LIVED EXPERIENCE OF DISABILITY

Damian Mellifont and
Jennifer Smith-Merry (Eds)

LIVED EXPERIENCE OF DISABILITY

Disability research and Australian disability policy

Disability Studies
Collection Editor
Damian Mellifont

LPP

First published in 2025 by Lived Places Publishing

British Library Cataloguing in Publication Data
A CIP record for this book is available from the British Library.

ISBN: 9781918026030 (pbk)
ISBN: 9781918026054 (ePDF)
ISBN: 9781918026047 (ePUB)

Cover design by Fiachra McCarthy
Book design by Rachel Trolove of Twin Trail Design
Typeset by Newgen Publishing, UK

Lived Places Publishing
P.O. Box 1845
47 Echo Avenue
Miller Place, NY 11764

www.livedplacespublishing.com

Abstract

This volume is informed by authors with lived experience of disability as well as genuine disability allies who hold a common passion towards making positive and practical differences in the lives of people with disability across Australia and further afield. It provides you with an opportunity to read and learn about lived experiences of disability together with their practical implications for future disability research and policy directions. Policy issue areas addressed in this book are wide-ranging and include those of codesign shortfalls, restrictive practices, linguistic and information deprivation, challenges confronting older people with dual sensory impairment, healthcare shortfalls in rural settings and the need for an increase in codesigned research in higher education and more broadly in policy design. Included in the volume are intriguing and timely research topics which hold strong potential to inform evidence-based disability policy in Australia as well as other places.

Key words

disability, policy, Australia, research, lived experience, inclusion

Contents

Content warning ix

Learning objectives x

Introduction 1

Chapter 1 Who has lived experience of disability? **11**

Chapter 2 What does 'good' disability policy look like? **37**

Chapter 3 Seeing the person before the problem: Using lived experience perspectives to eliminate restrictive practices **55**

Chapter 4 Policies to address information deprivation for people with disability **93**

Chapter 5 Epistemic gaps and policy absences: The plight of older people living with dual sensory impairment **121**

Chapter 6 Charcot-Marie-Tooth disease in rural Australia: A retrospective analysis of research and policy observation **161**

Chapter 7 The lived experience of neurodivergence in academic research studies: A neuro-affirming methodology **201**

Chapter 8 Towards a comprehensive research agenda: Fostering disability inclusion in research and innovation at the University of Queensland **235**

Discussion questions **265**

Recommended further reading **266**

Index **269**

Content warning

Readers are cautioned that this book contains references to and descriptions of violence, restrictive practices, suicidal ideation and disability discrimination. Readers are also advised that references to disability discrimination and restrictive practices are prevalent in Chapters 1 and 3, respectively.

Learning objectives

1. To understand the complexities and challenges in defining what counts as lived experience of disability.
2. To understand and explain the negative impacts of information accessibility gaps for people with disability.
3. To be able to explain why stakeholders with lived experience of disability need to be genuinely included in the codevelopment of disability policies in Australia and elsewhere.
4. To be able to describe some of the pressing disability issues in Australia that are yet to be recognised by policymakers.
5. To be able to identify some of the key barriers to including and valuing scholars with disability in Australian universities.
6. To be able to describe the various benefits that accompany disability research and broader policy that is codesigned and codeveloped with researchers with disability.

Introduction

Welcome to this exciting addition to the Disability Studies Collection. In the following chapters, you will read about lived experiences of disability together with their practical implications for future disability research and policy directions throughout Australia. We trust that you find these lived experiences of disability and related research and policy discussions to be engaging, educational and inspiring. This book is informed by authors with lived experience of disability as well as genuine disability allies who hold a common passion towards making positive and practical differences in the lives of people with disability across Australia and further afield. Please note that the first Editor will have more to say in relation to lived experience of disability in the chapter to follow where they delve deeply into this intriguing subject.

Why is the inclusion of lived experience of disability a central theme which binds the chapters of this book together? An appreciation and centring of the lived realities of any people's experiences are now increasingly fundamental to arguments which are supportive of self-determination and human rights (Bennett et al., 2024). Historically, people with disability have had limited involvement in redressing the disability policy issues which are key to their well-being (Ndlovu & Woldegiorgis, 2023). This is still the case and this gap continues to impact the way people with disability are included in society. There is much evidence supporting the role of stigma and discrimination towards excluding people with mental disability from employment, education and healthcare opportunities (Cummings et al., 2013; Evans-Lacko et al., 2012; Langmead, 2018). Yet, regardless of harmful disability stereotypes rarely impacting on people without disability, it is these persons who are often empowered to implement policy actions and decisions on behalf of the aforementioned population (Olsen, 2020). In a progressive development, the United Nations Convention on the Rights of Persons with Disabilities (UNCRPD) embraced a core principal that people with disability hold a fundamental right to be involved in the policies and decisions which affect them (Löve et al., 2017; Stein & Lord, 2010). By embracing this principal, the UNCRPD challenged a previously unrestrained norm in terms of who is included in disability policymaking (Löve, 2023). Specifically, Article 4(3) of this Convention requires governments to actively include people with disability in the development and implementation of disability policy and legislation (Löve et al., 2017). The rights of people with disability to be actively included and respected in disability policymaking activities therefore needs to be consistently acknowledged and enacted upon within Australia and beyond.

Advocacy has played a central role in promoting the inclusion of people with disability in disability policymaking. A right to participate in disability policymaking stems from the demands of people with disability to be treated as citizens who hold capacity to inform policy decisions and directions which impact upon their lives (Gunnarsdóttir & Löve, 2024; Quinn, 2009). This has been denied to people with disability in the past. As noted above, people with disability can hold shared experience of various forms of exclusion in society and the relevance of such experience to disability policymaking should not be downplayed. It is this shared experience which holds potential to build connections among people with disability, to progress meaningful engagement through this collective voice and to impact policy (D'Cruz et al., 2020; Veitch, 2024). Shared experience can act to inform not only pressing disability policy issues in employment, education and healthcare but also the measures that are urgently needed to redress them. Potential therefore exists for disability policymaking to be improved through having more people with disability who are not only qualified as policy professionals, but also who are qualified in terms of holding various lived experiences of disability (Mellifont & Smith-Merry, 2016). People with disability therefore need greater representation in codeveloping the policies that impact upon their lives as policymakers, and also as stakeholders who are included in welcoming and accessible disability policy consultations.

We the Editors of this volume hold a strong and shared appreciation for the importance of evidence-based disability policy that is informed by researchers with lived experience of disability and their allies. In putting together this volume we were motivated to have an open platform for people to present their perspectives on the inclusion of lived experience in policy in order to redress the gaps in current scholarship and policy design. Despite people with disability experiencing worse health than those without disability, various areas of disability policy interest remain under-researched (e.g. disability services and healthcare) (Krahn et al., 2015; Slattery et al., 2023). This indicates a need for greater government investment in disability policies whose issues and measures are informed by research that is either led by people with disability or codesigned with people with disability. Where disability studies are conducted, the inclusion of researchers with disability can vary from tokenistic inclusion right through to genuine inclusion as respected members of the research team (Bowers et al., 2008; Mellifont, 2023; Simpson, 2013). Smith-Merry et al. (2024) warned that the inclusion of researchers with disability risks falling away in the critical writing up of findings stage. By including lived experience of disability throughout the research process, power inequities can be challenged while the knowledge and expertise of the cohort to be most influenced by research findings is recognised (Chapman et al., 2024; Series, 2019). Conversely, exclusion of researchers with disability in studies about disability contributes to unequal opportunities for these researchers to be a part of knowledge production (including the academic careers that this knowledge production also supports), research that is not generalisable and ultimately poor disability policy outcomes (Ouellette, 2019; Rios et al., 2016; Slattery et al., 2023). Studies conducted with researchers with disability can require adjustments and accommodations, including access to assistive devices and other technologies; these are often not supported (or included) as part of research funding applications, which means that the knowledge of people who require support is also excluded (Watharow & Wayland, 2022). Consequently, the representation of researchers with lived experience of disability remains low where such accommodations for researchers with disabilities are needed (Bennett et al., 2024;

Mellifont et al., 2019). Unaccommodating disability research environments therefore need to be recognised and addressed as a disability policy priority.

We now provide a quick introduction to each of the following chapters. As mentioned above, in the upcoming chapter, the first Editor addresses the challenging question of who has lived experience of disability. Next, Jade McEwen critically discusses what 'good' disability policymaking codesign looks like. Bethany Easton and co-authors will then examine the pressing requirement to include lived experience perspectives in discourse concerning restrictive practices which confront people with disabilities. In their chapter, Cassandra Wright-Dole then draws on their lived experience of linguistic and information deprivation as well as scholarly evidence to call for recommendations to improve social and other outcomes for people with disability impacted by informational loss. Annmaree Watharow, Georgia Fagan and Moira Dunsmore discuss the importance of including the lived and living experiences of older persons with dual sensory impairment in disability policies and practices. Next, Scott Denton raises their policy observations, concerns and evidence-based ways forward regarding the pressing issue of experiences of Charcot-Marie-Tooth Disease in rural Australia. Jayne Garrod's chapter highlights the importance of participatory, insider, and codesigned research in terms of understanding the lived experiences of neurodivergent people. Last, Paul Harpur and colleagues investigate the University of Queensland's Champions of Change: Disability Inclusion Research and Innovation Plan in terms of its capacity to foster disability-inclusive research in higher education. Included among the chapters are suggested research topics which hold strong potential to inform evidence-based disability policy in Australia as well as other places. We conclude this text by offering learning objectives as well as a set of discussion questions for readers' careful consideration and responses.

Before going any further and reflecting our shared passion for disability research and disability policymaking, we would like to take this opportunity to offer our sincere thanks to the wonderful authors for their insightful and valuable contributions to this book. It was an honour and a pleasure to work with each of you in bringing this volume together. We would also like to thank the Lived Places Publishing cofounder, Mr David Parker, for his enthusiasm and support for not only this project, but also for the Disability Studies Collection more widely which we have both been enthusiastic champions of since its launch. We sincerely hope that you enjoy your reading journey into the lived experiences of disability as shared throughout this volume together with their implications for future disability research and policy directions in Australia and beyond.

Book Editors:

Dr Damian Mellifont

Lived Experience Postdoctoral Fellow and Associate Lecturer

Centre for Disability Research and Policy

The University of Sydney

Professor Jennifer Smith-Merry

ARC Industry Laureate Fellow

Centre for Disability Research and Policy

The University of Sydney

References

Bennett, J., Tattersall, A., McCormack, B., Moore, K., Mellifont, D., Wright, A. C., Fennis, L., Krayem, G., Sawan, M., & Huber, E. (2024). Illuminating lived experience: exploring researcher perspectives on co-design through participatory methods.

Bowers, L., Whittington, R., Nolan, P., Parkin, D., Curtis, S., Bhui, K., Hackney, D., Allan, T., & Simpson, A. (2008). Relationship between service ecology, special observation and self-harm during acute in-patient care: City-128 study. *The British Journal of Psychiatry, 193*(5), 395–401.

Chapman, K., Dixon, A., Kendall, E., & Clanchy, K. (2024). Defining dignity at the intersection of disability: a scoping review. *Disability and Rehabilitation*, *46*(23), 5404–5414.

Cummings, J. R., Lucas, S. M., & Druss, B. G. (2013). Addressing public stigma and disparities among persons with mental illness: The role of federal policy. *American journal of public health*, *103*(5), 781–785.

D'Cruz, K., Douglas, J., & Serry, T. (2020). Sharing stories of lived experience: A qualitative analysis of the intersection of experiences between storytellers with acquired brain injury and storytelling facilitators. *British Journal of Occupational Therapy*, *83*(9), 576–584.

Evans-Lacko, S., Brohan, E., Mojtabai, R., & Thornicroft, G. (2012). Association between public views of mental illness and self-stigma among individuals with mental illness in 14 European countries. *Psychological medicine*, *42*(8), 1741–1752.

Gunnarsdóttir, H. S.-o., & Löve, L. E. (2024). Rights in Crisis: Lived Experience as Knowledge in Policy Development During the COVID-19 Pandemic. *Scandinavian Journal of Disability Research*, *26*(1).

Krahn, G. L., Walker, D. K., & Correa-De-Araujo, R. (2015). Persons with disabilities as an unrecognized health disparity population. *American journal of public health*, *105*(S2), S198–S206.

Langmead, R. (2018). *The National Disability Insurance Scheme (NDIS) and mental health: A policy analysis* Murdoch University].

Löve, L., Traustadóttir, R., Quinn, G., & Rice, J. (2017). The inclusion of the lived experience of disability in policymaking. *Laws, 6*(4), 33.

Löve, L. E. (2023). Exclusion to inclusion: Lived experience of intellectual disabilities in national reporting on the CRPD. *Social Inclusion, 11*(2), 94–103.

Mellifont, D. (2023). A rapid review informing an assessment tool to support the inclusion of lived experience researchers in disability research. *Canadian Journal of Disability Studies, 12*(3), 86–109.

Mellifont, D., & Smith-Merry, J. (2016). Laying or delaying the groundwork? A critical framing analysis of Australia's National Disability Strategy from an implementation planning perspective. *Disability & Society, 31*(7), 929–947.

Mellifont, D., Smith-Merry, J., Dickinson, H., Llewellyn, G., Clifton, S., Ragen, J., Raffaele, M., & Williamson, P. (2019). The ableism elephant in the academy: A study examining academia as informed by Australian scholars with lived experience. *Disability & Society, 34*(7–8), 1180–1199.

Ndlovu, S., & Woldegiorgis, E. T. (2023). 'Nothing for us without us': Exclusion of students with disabilities in disability policy review at a South African institution of higher education. *African Journal of Teacher Education, 12*(1), 179–201.

Olsen, J. (2020). *Disability Unemployment in the UK: The Lived Experience of Disabling Barriers to Inclusion* Ulster University].

Ouellette, A. R. (2019). People with disabilities in human subjects research: A history of exploitation, a problem of exclusion. *Albany Law School Research Paper.*

Quinn, G. (2009). Resisting The" Temptation Of Elegance": Can The Convention On The Rights Of Persons With Disabilities Socialise

States To Right Behaviour? The UN convention on the rights of persons with disabilities,

Rios, D., Magasi, S., Novak, C., & Harniss, M. (2016). Conducting accessible research: including people with disabilities in public health, epidemiological, and outcomes studies. *American journal of public health, 106*(12), 2137–2144.

Series, L. (2019). Disability and human rights. *Routledge handbook of disability studies.*

Simpson, A. (2013). Setting up a mental health service user research group: A process paper. *Journal of Research in Nursing, 18*(8), 760–761.

Slattery, M., Ehrlich, C., Norwood, M., Amsters, D., & Allen, G. (2023). Disability research in Australia: Deciding to be a research participant and the experience of participation. *Journal of Empirical Research on Human Research Ethics, 18*(1–2), 37–49.

Smith-Merry, J., Darcy, S., Dew, A., Hemsley, B., Imms, C., O'Donovan, M.-A., Gallego, G., McVilly, K., Gilroy, J., & Carey, G. (2024). Who funds published disability research in Australia? *Journal of Disability Policy Studies*, 10442073241228840.

Stein, M. A., & Lord, J. E. (2010). Monitoring the Convention on the Rights of Persons with Disabilities: innovations, lost opportunities, and future potential. *Human Rights Quarterly, 32*(3), 689–728.

Veitch, H. P. H. (2024). *Disability and Transformation: Exploring the Lived Experiences of Students With Disabilities in South African Higher Education* Syracuse University].

Watharow, A., & Wayland, S. (2022). Making qualitative research inclusive: Methodological insights in disability research. *International Journal of Qualitative Methods, 21*, 16094069221095316.

1 Who has lived experience of disability?

Damian Mellifont

I acknowledge the Turrbal people as the traditional owners of the land upon which this chapter was written and I pay my respects to elders – past, present and emerging.

Introduction

I start with a quick introduction of myself and this chapter, including its aims, scope and structure. I also provide a few words regarding the choice of language style that is to be applied throughout my writing.

I am currently employed as a Lived Experience Postdoctoral Fellow and Lecturer with the Centre for Disability Research and Policy (CDRP) at the University of Sydney, Australia. I have been with the Centre since 2014 when I first joined in an Honorary Postdoctoral Fellow role. I am now a member of the CDRP leadership team that sets strategic direction for the Centre and very much enjoy my employment in an accommodating and inclusive environment. Such an environment does not just magically appear. This welcoming and safe workplace culture has been championed by the Centre's former Director and respected disability researcher and ally, Professor Jennifer Smith-Merry. An inclusive CDRP work environment stands in stark contrast to my prior work experiences in a policy role in the public service. It was in this inflexible government setting where my approved accommodations were inconsistently provided and where I would not openly disclose my neurodivergence for fear of discriminatory responses.

Having a formal medical diagnosis of obsessive-compulsive-disorder (OCD), I am neurodivergent. As a neurodivergent researcher, my lived experience-led and co-produced studies are designed to have positive and practical impacts on the lives of people with disability. These studies inform about redressing ableism (i.e. disability discrimination), together with practical and timely ways in which to advance the greater economic and social inclusion of people with disability. For example, a study that I led with Professor Jennifer Smith-Merry and Dr Kim Bulkeley on the policy issue of disability employment (specifically the under-representation of employees with lived experience of disability across Australian Disability Services) revealed that only half of these service organisations have at least one employee with disability and less than a quarter (24%) of organisations have a board member with disability (Mellifont et al., 2023). Highlighting the policy relevance and timeliness of our study, this research informed questioning at Public Hearing 32 of the Royal Commission into the Violence, Abuse, Neglect and Exploitation of people with disability held in Brisbane from 13 to 17 February 2023. More broadly, my research advocacy efforts support the disability inclusion mantra of 'nothing about us without us' to be widely applied across disability research and policy settings in Australia and elsewhere.

I now commence this chapter by addressing the thought-provoking question of who has lived experience of disability? My response to this question is to be informed by a critical examination of scholarly constructions of lived experience of disability, together with their complexities and practical implications. Next, I critically discuss the topic of representations of lived expertise in disability research and disability policy spaces. I then build an evidence-based case for including more people with lived experience of disability in codesigned and co-produced disability research and policymaking activities. I conclude my chapter by providing readers with a summary of avenues for future research relating to the intriguing question of 'who has lived experience'?

Before this chapter gets underway, some quick words in relation to the disability language that is to be applied. Person-first language reflects the social model of disability where people are positioned before their disability (e.g. researcher with disability) (Disabled People's Organisations Australia, 2022). The social model of disability and its support for a removal of barriers to social inclusion and the introduction of anti-discrimination law stands in contrast to the medical model and its medicalisation of people with lived experience of disability (Linton, 1998; Shakespeare, 2006). I purposefully use person-first language in the writing of this chapter. And while I choose to identify as neurodivergent rather than a person with OCD, I do not expect others to follow my personal choice. That is to say, I respect the rights and freedoms of others to choose how they prefer to identify.

Scholarly constructions of lived experience of disability, complexities and practical implications

Now, onto the question of who has lived experience of disability? Noting the complex nature of this question, I start by recognising that the language of lived experience is open to construction with no fixed meaning available (Byrne, 2013; Mellifont & Smith-Merry, 2021). In terms of lived experience of disability, it needs to be realised that everyone has lived experience but not everyone has lived experience of disability such as mental ill health (Morgan & Lawson, 2015; Smith, 2014). Disability allies are included among this latter group. Woodard et al. (2012) noted the importance of disability allies as faculty champions in the academy. Allies can thus lay claim to holding lived experience in providing valuable disability allyships, as expressed in educational settings in this instance. These experiences, however, do not extend to the personal challenges that many staff and students with disability experience on and off campus. Prominent among these challenges is ableism (i.e. disability discrimination) (Mellifont, 2023; Mellifont et al., 2019). While there exists a 'uniqueness' to an individual's lived experience (Bennet et al., 2024, p. 9), shared insights can accompany direct experiences with dismissal and discounting (Byrne, 2017; Duvnjak et al., 2022). These are deep and intimate constructions that cannot be attained from simply reading about or observing discrimination as experienced by people with disability. Understanding can at times be difficult to put into words given the hurt, trauma and emotions involved.

Gaps in understanding as well as misrepresentations of disability are readily found in the field of disability care. Carers can be said to have lived experience of caring for people with disability. However, if a carer does not have a disability, the same individual cannot justifiably or ethically lay claim to having lived experience of disability. Rieck et al. (2019) captured the complexities of a mother who provided care for a young adult with an intellectual disability. It needs to be recognised however that this particular individual's lived experiences are different to the lived experiences of the person with intellectual disability for whom they care. Acknowledging the challenging and often times uncompensated work that many carers regularly carry out, respect for lived experience of disability is nevertheless needed to avoid misrepresentation. In this light, Chapman, Dixon, Kendall, et al. (2024, p. 2) explicitly stated in their methods 'to ensure that the scoping literature review was grounded in the perspectives of lived experience of disability, the authorship team was formed to include a senior academic (EK) who is a family member of people with disability and has personal experience of a degenerative disabling health condition'. Helping to explain this intersectionality, this particular senior scholar is exposed not only to their lived experience of disability, but also to the experience of having family members with disability.

Closely aligning to queries about who has lived experience of disability is the question of who holds expertise? Lived expertise is defined as 'knowledge, insights, understanding and wisdom gathered through lived experience' (Sandhu, 2017, p. 5). So, while lived experience can be thought of as raw experiences, lived expertise is the knowledge that comes from reflecting on these experiences (Cataldo et al., 2021). Hence, accompanying lived experiences of disability such as mental ill health is a level of expertise that cannot otherwise be rightfully claimed, and this expertise along with the voices of people with disability need to be privileged, respected and valued (Byrne & Wykes, 2020; Chapman, Dixon, Ehrlich, et al., 2024; Mellifont, 2019). For instance, peer researchers' insider expertise as gained through their lived experiences of homelessness successfully informed a study on this topic (Elliott et al., 2002; Massie et al., 2018). One does not have to search too far, however, to identify instances where respect for and representations of lived expertise is deficient or missing altogether. Gibbs (2022) made the observation that while many with lived experience are often the experts (e.g. academics, professionals), they rarely are positioned with the so-called experts who maintain power. While leaders without disability and their achievements in disability research and policy spaces need to be recognised and appreciated, it is the ethical leader without disability who is prepared to have power fairly redistributed with people who have relevant lived expertise and professional qualifications (or the capacity to develop professional expertise through training). It is noteworthy however that there exists no training in the world that can successfully provide lived expertise of disability to leaders without disability.

Remaining cognisant of the above-mentioned possibilities for misrepresentation and the protection of power bases, there are no set criteria that can be neatly applied to define what counts as lived experience of disability. Strong arguments are made against any direction or efforts towards the development of this criteria. Roennfeldt and Byrne (2020) posed the puzzling question of what counts as lived experience and what level or amount of lived experience is counted as 'enough'? In addition to this questioning, any attempts to develop and rigidly apply criteria to lived experience of disability is to risk dismissing individual differences by forcing people to justify themselves (Voronka, 2016; Waddingham, 2021). Complicating matters even further, organisational recruiters have expressed biases with preferences voiced for less disordered forms of disability, with lived experience of mental illness falling outside of what is considered 'a socially acceptable disability type' in many cultures (Bakhshi et al., 2006, p. 25; Waddingham, 2021). Anderson and Bigby (2023) also questioned the transferability of lived experience on occasions where boards of organisations that support people with intellectual disabilities engage individuals with lived experiences of sensory or physical disabilities. It should therefore not be assumed that lived experience of a particular disability somehow magically transfers into the holding of expertise in another disability type.

With multiple and at times competing constructions of lived experience, disability policymakers need to apply caution when engaging in related lively discussions which can and do ensue. According to Jones et al. (2021), debates about terminology, including that of lived experience, can act as a distraction from the significant policy issues at hand and where people with disability continue to be under-represented in policy activities. Activities that are key to informing about the disability challenges to be raised in the first place and subsequently how these issues are to be addressed (or, aligning with the satisficing model and reflecting the realities of policymaking, reduced). I have witnessed occasions on social media where individuals attempt to position their constructions of lived experience of disability as correct and unquestionable, while at the same time publicly disrespecting and demeaning the constructions of others. Upon reading such negative social media commentary, I cannot help but think that this energy would be better served in collaborative efforts to expose and address the common enemy of people with disability; this enemy being ableism (i.e. disability discrimination).

So far in this chapter, I have referred to *lived experience of disability* which implies reflections on or descriptions of past experiences with disability. Studies have, however, made mention of *living experience with disability* to capture various present happenings (e.g. the masking of disability, experiences of bullying etc.) (Anika, 2021; Dillaway et al., 2022). This highlights the appropriateness of language capturing disability experiences happening in the now in addition to those experiences which have passed. This brings us to future tense and *yet to be lived experiences of disability*. With around 15% of the world's population with lived experience of disability, this percentage is rising as people age (United Nations, 2024). 'Yet to be' lived experiences of disability is thus a growing policy issue for policymakers in Australia and elsewhere.

Appreciating the aforementioned complexities surrounding who has lived experience of disability as well as the timings of these experiences, freedom of choice in expressing lived experiences (e.g. experiences associated with madness, neurodivergence, survival, disorder, disability etc) is needed. Individuals can flexibly identify with one or more terms (e.g. mad, neurodivergent, survivor, disordered, person with disability) or other descriptors and at different times. From my perspective and as noted in my introduction, I identify as neurodivergent on the proviso that my approved accommodations are *consistently* in place. One such accommodation is that my presentations are performed in an asynchronous manner (i.e. these presentations are pre-recorded with questions taken on notice). Take this approved and reasonable accommodation away, as has happened on multiple occasions while employed in the public service, and I identify as a person with disability.

Representations of lived experience of disability in disability research and disability policy spaces

Representations of lived experience of disability in research about disability occurs at varying levels. At the highest level of inclusion is lived experience-led studies, with codesigned and co-produced research positioned at the preceding level (Bellingham et al., 2023). Researchers with lived experience of disability can therefore lead or colead studies and involve research team members with or without this experience. Within the research-led approach, the study aims, collection methods and all other decisions remain in the control of researchers with lived experience (Bennet et al., 2024). It is at this highest level of inclusion where researchers with lived experience are given opportunities to demonstrate their leadership and research skills across the entire disability research project. So, how might a lived experience led study play out in practice? Dr Annmaree Watharow and I co-led a study where we investigated our respective lived experiences as deafblind and neurodivergent (Watharow & Mellifont, 2024). To our knowledge, this was the world's first qualitative, co-led study by a deafblind researcher and a neurodivergent researcher. The study was conducted in a respectful, flexible and cooperative way, allowing for our differing accommodation needs (e.g. large font size, written responses to interview questions) to be consistently met. Recognising the limitation of a small case study, our research was nevertheless practical, in that we successfully delivered a lived experience informed roadmap towards inclusive research design. This roadmap offered practical directions for accommodating deafblind and neurodivergent researchers and developing and supporting research career pathways (Watharow & Mellifont, 2024).

Also representing a strong level of involvement, codesigned or co-produced research is defined in terms of collaboratively constructing knowledge and engaging with stakeholders, including service users and carers (Greenhalgh et al., 2016; Halvorsrud et al., 2021; Voronka, 2016). Codesign involves forming collaborative partnerships and creatively *working with* people with various lived experiences (Borzenkova et al., 2023; Labattaglia, 2019). The literature, however, cautioned that co-production with researchers with lived experience can be inconsistently applied in practice (Durose et al., 2022; Smith et al., 2023). Legitimate codesigned and co-produced disability research therefore transcends empty rhetoric and 'tick a box' approaches to genuinely include researchers with lived experience of disability. Codesigned research is about *inclusive action* rather than repeated words about inclusion. I can recall attending an online conference where one of the presenters raised the important topic of codesign. However, codesign was repeated so many times over the course of their presentation that some online attendees started to play a game of buzzword bingo in the chat. Terms such as codesign and co-production should not be reduced to buzzwords that hold no practical application. Nor should they be flippantly thrown about in unconvincing attempts to appear inclusive of people with lived experience of disability. In contrast, co-production embraces the principle of authentically including people with lived experience in conducting studies as coresearchers while maintaining equitable partnerships throughout the research journey (Facer et al., 2016; Nectoux et al., 2023; Smith et al., 2023; Whitburn & Goodley, 2022).

Over the last 20 years in a shift towards social justice, co-production has brought together people with lived experience of disability into studies with disability researchers (Anderson, 2023; Gray, 2023). Recognising this progress, there continues to be a shortage of people with disability included in disability research following an undervaluing of lived expertise (Banas et al., 2019; Mellifont et al., 2019). With professional expertise at times elevated above lived experience expertise, academic structures and systems are at risk of dismissing expertise by experience (David et al., 2023; Mahboub et al., 2023). Inclusive academic structures value lived expertise while at the same time encouraging supportive and accommodating research settings. It is in these inclusive environments where people with lived experience of disability can be supported in developing their research skills (where such skills development is needed, recognising that many researchers with lived experience of disability are PhD qualified) and contribute to disability studies to their greatest capacity. In this way, people with lived experience of disability are not set up to fail as researchers or unfairly treated in tokenistic ways throughout the disability research process. Rather, they are authentically included in research teams, matched to roles and pay grades commensurate with their goals, skills and abilities and provided with accessible training opportunities to develop research expertise (again, wherever needed).

Researchers who continue to conduct studies *about* disability and who refuse to include researchers *with* lived experience of disability are opening themselves to questions about the quality of their studies. For instance, the inclusion of lived experience in disability research offers perspectives that are not available to teams lacking in this experience (e.g. perspectives about disability employment) (Fraser-Barbour et al., 2023). Disability research teams with no lived experience are also at risk of perpetuating negative disability stereotypes where a medical model-driven deficit focus of disability can dominate. Autistic researcher and professor Nick Walker cautioned about controversial and abusive conversion therapy techniques continuing to be carelessly published in academic journals (Walker & Raymaker, 2021; Yergeau, 2018). A need therefore exists to shift away from disability studies that feed discriminatory messages (e.g. people having to be cured of their neurodivergence). Supporting this shift, Smith-Merry et al. (2024) cautioned about the prospect of lived experience becoming only partially included in the research process (i.e. this experience not extending to stages of manuscript writing and scholarly publication). The exclusion of lived experience in these critical final stages of research risks ableist manuscript content being overlooked, particularly on occasions where lived experience is also absent among manuscript reviewers. Yet another pressing research question thus becomes, who has lived expertise among disability manuscript reviewers? Chief editors of disability journals are therefore challenged to ensure that lived experience of disability is represented among their reviewers.

I now move the discussion on to representations of lived experience of disability in disability policymaking. In accordance with the UNCRPD Article 4(3), government policy needs to be codesigned and include the voices of people with lived experience of disability (Löve et al., 2017; Nally et al., 2022). The inclusion of lived experience of disability in shaping disability policies and services is thus critical to the advancement of human rights and equity (Anderson & Bigby, 2023; Malbon et al., 2024). Rieger (2020) too called for disability policy, services and programmes to be codesigned with people with lived experience. The main goal of codesigned policy is to co-create tailored solutions to issues (e.g. housing insecurity/homelessness) by applying the expertise of individuals who have lived experiences with the issues under investigation (Constantine, 2023; Labattaglia et al., 2023; Meltzer et al., 2021; Robinson et al., 2024). Goldstraw (2021) too noted the importance of purposefully listening to the voices of people with lived experience in the making of policies that directly impact upon their lives. Despite the UN, scholarly and advocacy support for inclusive disability policymaking, significant forms of resistance persist. Power imbalances continue where government and political agents decide upon what policy content is informed through stakeholder consultations and without any accountability for their decisions (Löve, 2023). Furthermore, a greater representation of people with disability across the policy development process can reduce control and power for some, with marginalised groups advocating for their greater engagement in policy agenda setting and activities (Disability Advocacy Network Australia, 2012; Löve et al., 2017). Care is therefore needed in disability policymaking in Australia and elsewhere to avoid an under-representation of lived experience and 'fake' codesign. According to Mladenov (2023), this disingenuous form of policymaking attempts to legitimise an inequitable status quo through a refusal to redistribute power, with inequity maintained through various soft forms of power control (e.g. hiding information, speaking in policy jargon and nudging people to move in certain directions).

Building an evidence-based case for including more people with lived experience of disability in disability research and policymaking

Informed by the above discussion, the case for a greater inclusion of lived experience of disability in disability research and policymaking activities is a strong one. To begin with, including lived experience in research design enables the exploration of topics that are of particular relevance to disability communities (Strnadová et al., 2022). In addition to informing where the research is heading, the inclusion of lived experience researchers brings 'insider knowledge' that eludes researchers without disability (Mellifont et al., 2019; Watharow & Wayland, 2022). The value of having ready access to established, trusted and extensive disability networks should also not be dismissed or downplayed. For it is this lived experience of disability which can enable contact with study populations that might otherwise remain out of reach as well as helping to comprehend the important messages that study participants with disability are communicating (Biringer et al., 2016; Elliott et al., 2002).

Co-produced studies empower researchers with lived experience of disability (Lombard-Vance et al., 2023). Empowerment in terms of people with disability taking back power (or refusing to acknowledge illegitimately held power) is signified in many ways. For example, neurodivergent voices reflective of lived experience challenge studies which promote questionable 'treatments', including sensory desensitisation and early intervention by positioning these approaches as forms of abuse (Shaw et al., 2022). The neurodivergent voices of those who have lived experiences of these kinds of abusive treatments should never be silenced by those without these experiences (e.g. politicians, policymakers, carers, researchers or healthcare professionals who carry out these treatments and who might have vested financial interests in their unabated continuation).

Co-produced policy also empowers people with disability through a sharing of authority and the valuing of knowledge that comes from lived experience while practically applying this knowledge to inform disability policy (Martin et al., 2022; Smith, 2022). More people with lived experience of disability need to take power and be drivers of disability policy direction, both as policymakers and valued stakeholders. It is easy for governments to dismiss, gaslight and label stakeholders with lived experience of disability and who publicly criticise disability policy directions as scaremongers or 'unstable' conspiracy theorists. But these kinds of dismissals are ableist, in that they fail to give any real consideration to the possible validity of the concerns raised. Rather, the voices of people with lived experience of disability need to be heard in relation to complex policy issues and pragmatically acted upon through co-produced measures (Hoogendam, 2023; Patrick et al., 2022; Peters, 2023).

Genuinely inclusive and respectful disability policymaking is possible. Co-produced policy has been successfully applied across diverse fields, including healthcare access, disaster risk reduction for people with disability and disability employment (Bishop et al., 2023; Khayatzadeh-Mahani et al., 2020; Yamori, 2020). However, while these texts offer sound examples of inclusive policymaking, it would be naïve to assume that co-produced disability policy is the norm rather than the exception.

A summary of avenues for future research relating to the question of 'who has lived experience of disability'?

To follow is a list of research topics relating to the question of 'who has lived experience of disability'? (see Box 1). This includes topics that endeavour to inform ways of decreasing misrepresentations of lived experience of disability and increasing representations of people with disability in disability research and policymaking teams. Aligning with messages of inclusion (made throughout this chapter), such future research needs to be either lived experience-led by or codesigned with people with disability.

Box 1: 'Who has lived experience of disability'? related avenues of research.

1. To what extent are people (e.g. carers) without disability misrepresenting themselves and applying for positions (including disability research and policy positions) which are advertised for applicants who hold lived experience of disability?
2. To what degree are leaders without disability in disability research and policymaking spaces prepared to have power fairly redistributed with people who have lived experience of disability and professional expertise?
3. To what extent are social media debates about who qualifies as having lived experience of disability acting as distractions from addressing pressing disability policy issues (e.g. disability unemployment)?
4. How well are Australian disability policymakers forecasting and planning for 'yet to be lived experiences' of disability and how does this compare against policy efforts of other nations?
5. What is the magnitude of the policy issue whereby disability studies are claimed to be codesigned with researchers with lived experience of disability but are not in practice?
6. What are the forms of resistance to exclusionary disability research and policymaking and how do these measures compare in terms of their effectiveness?
7. To what extent are the concerns of stakeholders who have lived experience of disability and of the disability policy issues at hand (e.g. disability unemployment) unfairly dismissed by policymakers without disability?

Conclusion

In this chapter, I have critically discussed scholarly constructions of lived experience of disability as well as their complexities and practical implications. I have also critically examined who has lived experience in disability research and disability policy spaces. Last, I have revealed an evidence-based case for including more people with lived experience of disability in disability research and policymaking activities. I hope this chapter has provided readers with much food for thought on the multifaceted, intriguing and complex question of who has lived experience of disability? Despite the complexities raised, three words remain crystal clear in my take-home message – 'avoid fake representation'. So, if you are a carer without disability, do not misrepresent yourself as having lived experience of disability. If you are a leader in a disability research or policy space and do not have a disability, do not put yourself forward as having lived experience of disability. To do so is to not only mispresent yourself, but to also show disrespect towards the people who have this lived experience. Finally, I trust that I've offered some interesting research pathways related to the question of 'who has lived experience of disability'? that once travelled, will inform a range of pressing disability policy issues.

References

Anderson, S. (2023). Threats to valuing diverse voices in public debates about disability. A case study from social media. *Research and Practice in Intellectual and Developmental Disabilities, 10*(1), 48–60.

Anderson, S., & Bigby, C. (2023). 'Nothing about us without us'. Including Lived Experiences of People with Intellectual Disabilities in Policy and Service Design. *Disability Practice: Safeguarding Quality Service Delivery*, 225–246.

Anika, A. S. (2021). *Understanding the patterns of bullying and it's mental health effects among the youth with physical disability in Bangladesh* Bangladesh Health Professions Institute, Faculty of Medicine, the University ...].

Bakhshi, P., Trani, J.-F., & Rolland, C. (2006). Conducting surveys on disability: A comprehensive toolkit.

Banas, J. R., Magasi, S., The, K., & Victorson, D. E. (2019). Recruiting and retaining people with disabilities for qualitative health research: Challenges and solutions. *Qualitative Health Research*, *29*(7), 1056–1064.

Bellingham, B., Elder, E., Foxlewin, B., Gale, N., Rose, G., Sam, K., Thorburn, K., & River, J. (2023). Co-design kickstarter.

Bennet, J., Tattersall, A., McCormack, B., Moore, K., Mellifont, D., Conley Wright, A., Fennis, L., Krayem, G., Sawan, M., Huber, E., O'Callaghan, M., & Country, G. (2024). *Illuminating Lived Experience Exploring Researcher Perspectives on Co-design Through Participatory Methods*. The University of Sydney.

Biringer, E., Davidson, L., Sundfør, B., Ruud, T., & Borg, M. (2016). Experiences of support in working toward personal recovery goals: a collaborative, qualitative study. *BMC psychiatry*, *16*, 1–14.

Bishop, G. M., Llewellyn, G., Kavanagh, A. M., Badland, H., Bailie, J., Stancliffe, R., Emerson, E., Fortune, N., & Aitken, Z. (2023). Disability-related inequalities in the prevalence of loneliness across the lifespan: trends from Australia, 2003 to 2020.

Borzenkova, G., Tang, J., & Niedderer, K. (2023). Co-designing with children with cerebral palsy: context and co-design principles.

Byrne, L. (2013). *A grounded theory study of lived experience mental health practitioners within the wider workforce* CQUniversity].

Byrne, L. (2017). *Promoting Lived Experience Perspective: Discussion Paper*. Queensland Mental Health Commission.

Byrne, L., & Wykes, T. (2020). A role for lived experience mental health leadership in the age of Covid-19. *Journal of Mental Health, 29*(3), 243-246.

Cataldo, M. L., Street, B., Rynehart, S., White, C., & Larsen, K. (2021). Remembering radical roots: Lived experience participation movements and the risks and responsibilities of co-design in community-led change. *Parity, 34*(6), 13–16.

Chapman, K., Dixon, A., Ehrlich, C., & Kendall, E. (2024). Dignity and the Importance of Acknowledgement of Personhood for People With Disability. *Qualitative Health Research, 34*(1–2), 141–153.

Chapman, K., Dixon, A., Kendall, E., & Clanchy, K. (2024). Defining dignity at the intersection of disability: a scoping review. *Disability and rehabilitation*, 1–11.

Constantine, S. (2023). Consumer participation in homelessness service delivery in Australia: What is it for? *Australian Journal of Social Issues.*

David, C., Johnson, B., & Ramcharan, P. (2023). NDIS partnership working? Paradoxes, contested spaces and aspirations of disability leaders, family carers and disability services. *Australian Journal of Social Issues.*

Dillaway, H. E., James, A. J., & Horn, A. J. (2022). The Invisibilities of Disability: Compiling Conversations. *Sociation, 21*(1).

Disability Advocacy Network Australia. (2012). *Submission National Disability Strategy 2010–2020: Laying the Groundwork (2011–2014)*. DANA.

Disabled People's Organisations Australia. (2022). *Terminology.* https://dpoa.org.au/about/terminology/

Durose, C., Perry, B., & Richardson, L. (2022). Is co-production a 'good'concept? Three responses. *Futures, 142*, 102999.

Duvnjak, A., Stewart, V., Young, P., & Turvey, L. (2022). How does lived experience of incarceration impact upon the helping process in social work practice?: A scoping review. *The British Journal of Social Work, 52*(1), 354–373.

Elliott, E., Watson, A. J., & Harries, U. (2002). Harnessing expertise: involving peer interviewers in qualitative research with hard-to-reach populations. *Health Expectations, 5*(2), 172–178.

Facer, K., Enright, B., & Dunleavy, K. (2016). *The 'public value' of research: creating long-term conversations between universities and communities* https://www.bristol.ac.uk/media-library/sites/policybristol/briefings-and-reports-pdfs/pre-2017-briefings--reports-pdfs/PolicyBristol_Report_08_2016_universities_communities_conversations.pdf

Fraser-Barbour, E., Robinson, S., Gendera, S., Burton-Clark, I., Fisher, K. R., Alexander, J., & Howe, K. (2023). Shifting power to people with disability in co-designed research. *Disability & society*, 1–22.

Gibbs, E. (2022). *Lived expertise mean sexperts*. http://elgibbs.com.au/lived-expertise-means-experts/

Goldstraw, K. (2021). "Why aren't we heard with our voices?" APLE Collective's lived experience of poverty. In *Socially Distanced Activism* (pp. 11–30). Policy Press.

Gray, B. (2023). Lived experience research: a guide to the barriers and facilitators from a service user's perspective. *Psychosis*, 1–5.

Greenhalgh, T., Jackson, C., Shaw, S., & Janamian, T. (2016). Achieving research impact through co-creation in community-based health services: literature review and case study. *The Milbank Quarterly, 94*(2), 392–429.

Halvorsrud, K., Kucharska, J., Adlington, K., Rüdell, K., Brown Hajdukova, E., Nazroo, J., Haarmans, M., Rhodes, J., & Bhui, K. (2021). Identifying evidence of effectiveness in the co-creation of research: a systematic review and meta-analysis of the international healthcare literature. *Journal of public health, 43*(1), 197–208.

Hoogendam, R. (2023). *Reacting to the Rise in Accountability Requirements: A Case Study of Status of Women Canada's Women's Program* Carleton University.

Jones, N., Atterbury, K., Byrne, L., Carras, M., Brown, M., & Phalen, P. (2021). Lived experience, research leadership, and the transformation of mental health services: building a researcher pipeline. *Psychiatric Services, 72*(5), 591–593.

Khayatzadeh-Mahani, A., Wittevrongel, K., Petermann, L., Graham, I. D., & Zwicker, J. D. (2020). Stakeholders' engagement in co-producing policy-relevant knowledge to facilitate employment for persons with developmental disabilities. *Health research policy and systems, 18*, 1–17.

Labattaglia, O. (2019). *Accessible Co-design* Auckland University of Technology].

Labattaglia, O., Reay, S., & Nakarada-Kordic, I. (2023). Co-designing accessible co-design. *Design for Health*, 1–17.

Linton, S. (1998). Disability studies/not disability studies. *Disability & society, 13*(4), 525–539.

Lombard-Vance, R., Soye, E., Ferri, D., McEvoy, E., MacLachlan, M., & Sarlio-Siintola, S. (2023). Applying the 'human rights model of disability' to informed consent: Experiences and reflections from the SHAPES project. *Disabilities, 3*(1), 28–47.

Löve, L., Traustadóttir, R., Quinn, G., & Rice, J. (2017). The inclusion of the lived experience of disability in policymaking. *Laws, 6*(4), 33.

Löve, L. E. (2023). Exclusion to Inclusion: Lived Experience of Intellectual Disabilities in National Reporting on the CRPD. *Social Inclusion, 11*(2), 94–103.

Mahboub, L., Martin, R., & Hodgson, D. (2023). A program for valuing mental health lived experience in social work education. *Australian Social Work, 76*(4), 441–454.

Malbon, E., Meltzer, A., & Carey, G. (2024). The NDIS at ten years: designing an equitable scheme for the next decade. *The Medical Journal of Australia*, *220*(1), 55–55.

Martin, R. A., Baker, A. P., Smiler, K., Middleton, L., Hay-Smith, J., Kayes, N., Grace, C., Apiata, T. A. M., Nunnerley, J. L., & Brown, A. E. (2022). Flourishing together: research protocol for developing methods to better include disabled people's knowledge in health policy development. *BMC Health Services Research*, *22*(1), 1–12.

Massie, R., Machin, R., McCormack, F., & Kurth, J. (2018). Having a voice: A collaborative research project exploring the challenges and assets of people experiencing homelessness. *Journal of Integrated Care*, *26*(4), 342–352.

Mellifont, D. (2019). Non-disabled space invaders! A study critically exploring the scholarly reporting of research attributes for persons with and without disability. *Studies in Social Justice*, *13*(2), 304–321.

Mellifont, D. (2023). Ableist ivory towers: A narrative review informing about the lived experiences of neurodivergent staff in contemporary higher education. *Disability & society*, *38*(5), 865–886.

Mellifont, D., & Smith-Merry, J. (2021). *Disability, Identity, and Language Choices: Person-first, identity-first, and beyond*. https://livedplacespublishing.com/blog/disability-identity-and-language-choices-person-first-identity-first-and-beyond

Mellifont, D., Smith-Merry, J., Dickinson, H., Llewellyn, G., Clifton, S., Ragen, J., Raffaele, M., & Williamson, P. (2019). The ableism elephant in the academy: A study examining academia as informed by Australian scholars with lived experience. *Disability & society*, *34*(7–8), 1180–1199.

Mellifont, D., Smith-Merry, J., & Bulkeley, K. (2023). The employment of people with lived experience of disability in Australian disability services. *Social Policy & Administration*, *57*(5), 642–655.

Meltzer, A., Dickinson, H., Malbon, E., & Carey, G. (2021). Why is lived experience important for market stewardship? A proposed framework for why and how lived experience should be included in stewarding disability markets. *Evidence & Policy*, *17*(2), 335–347.

Mladenov, T. (2023). Co-production. 'A European Framework for Social Services of Excellence for Persons with Disabilities'-a workshop organised by ENIL,

Morgan, P., & Lawson, J. (2015). Developing guidelines for sharing lived experience of staff in health and social care. *Mental Health and Social Inclusion*, *19*(2), 78–86.

Nally, D., Moore, S. S., & Gowran, R. J. (2022). How governments manage personal assistance schemes in response to the United Nations Convention on the Rights of Persons with Disabilities: A Scoping Review. *Disability & society*, *37*(10), 1728–1751.

Nectoux, S., Magee, L., & Soldatic, K. (2023). Sensing technologies, digital inclusion, and disability diversity. *Journal of Computer-Mediated Communication*, *28*(5), zmad026.

Patrick, R., Garthwaite, K., Power, M., Kaufman, J., Page, G., Pybus, K., Warnock, R., Aldridge, H., Flew, L., & Lee, T. (2022). Covid realities documenting life on a low income during the pandemic. *Nuffield Foundation*.

Peters, L. A. (2023). Embracing neurodiversity to enhance the post-graduate researcher experience: Reflections from a doctoral student. *Fields: journal of Huddersfield student research*, *1*(1).

Rieck, M., Shakespeare-Finch, J., Märtsin, M., & Knox, M. (2019). The lived experience of a mother of a young adult with intellectual disability:'my Daughter as my Enlightenment'. *Scandinavian Journal of Disability Research*, *21*(1), 49–57.

Rieger, J. (2020). Right to participate: Co-Designing disability policies in Australia. *QUT Centre for Justice Briefing Papers*(12), 1–4.

Robinson, S., Idle, J., Fisher, K. R., Reedy, K., Newman, C., Purcal, C., Giuntoli, G., Byrne, S., Nankivell, R., & Burner, G. (2024). How do self-advocates use community development to change attitudes to disability? *British Journal of Learning Disabilities*, *52*(1), 87–100.

Roennfeldt, H., & Byrne, L. (2020). How much 'lived experience' is enough? Understanding mental health lived experience work from a management perspective. *Australian Health Review*, *44*(6), 898–903.

Sandhu, B. (2017). The value of lived experience in social change. *Available at: thelivedexperience. org [accessed 28 Nov 2018].*

Shakespeare, T. (2006). The social model of disability. *The disability studies reader*, *2*(3), 197–204.

Shaw, C., Churchill, V., Curtain, S., Davies, A., Davis, B., Kalenderidis, Z., Hunt, E. L., McKenzie, B., Murray, M., & Thompson, G. A. (2022). Lived Experience Perspectives on Ableism Within and Beyond Music Therapists' Professional Identities. *Music Therapy Perspectives*, *40*(2), 143–151.

Smith-Merry, J., Darcy, S., Dew, A., Hemsley, B., Imms, C., O'Donovan, M.-A., Gallego, G., McVilly, K., Gilroy, J., & Carey, G. (2024). Who Funds Published Disability Research in Australia? *Journal of Disability Policy Studies*, 10442073241228840.

Smith, B., Williams, O., Bone, L., & Collective, t. M. S. W. C.-p. (2023). Co-production: A resource to guide co-producing research in the sport, exercise, and health sciences. *Qualitative Research in Sport, Exercise and Health*, *15*(2), 159–187.

Smith, H. (2014). How Has Activism Impacted Theory Development? An Exploration of the Addiction and Disability Fields. *Unpublished MA thesis, York University.*

Smith, S. R. (2022). Conclusion: The Human Condition, Conflicting Experiences of Time, Emotion and Self-Consciousness, and Value Incommensurability. In *The Ontology of Well-Being in Social Policy and Welfare Practice* (pp. 225–260). Springer.

Strnadová, I., Dowse, L., & Garcia-Lee, B. (2022). Doing research inclusively: Co-production in action.

United Nations. (2024). *Factsheet on persons with disabilities.* https://www.un.org/development/desa/disabilities/resources/factsheet-on-persons-with-disabilities.html

Voronka, J. (2016). The politics of 'people with lived experience' Experiential authority and the risks of strategic essentialism. *Philosophy, Psychiatry, & Psychology, 23*(3), 189–201.

Waddingham, R. (2021). *Lived Experience Leadership.* https://www.nsun.org.uk/wp-content/uploads/2021/11/LEL-Report-Nov-2021.pdf

Walker, N., & Raymaker, D. M. (2021). Toward a neuroqueer future: An interview with Nick Walker. *Autism in Adulthood, 3*(1), 5–10.

Watharow, A., & Mellifont, D. (2024). A case study unveiling challenges and supports for deafblind and neurodivergent researchers and participants. *Journal of Humanity and Social Justice.,* 109–123.

Watharow, A., & Wayland, S. (2022). Making qualitative research inclusive: Methodological insights in disability research. *International Journal of Qualitative Methods, 21,* 16094069221095316.

Whitburn, B., & Goodley, D. (2022). Storying disability's potential. *International journal of inclusive education, 26*(4), 415–428.

Woodard, L. J., Havercamp, S. M., Zwygart, K. K., & Perkins, E. A. (2012). An innovative clerkship module focused on patients with disabilities. *Academic medicine, 87*(4), 537–542.

Yamori, K. (2020). *Disaster Risk Communication.* Springer.

Yergeau, M. R. (2018). *Authoring autism: On rhetoric and neurological queerness.* Duke University Press.

2
What does 'good' disability policy look like?

Jade McEwen

Introduction

Disability policy is a term used to describe documented principles of action, which typically aim to ensure the rights and inclusion of people with disability. In Australia, disability policy is normally written by three main actors: Commonwealth Government, state and territory governments and by organisations responsible for supporting people with disability. Broadly, the focus of disability policy is to ensure equal rights, opportunity and inclusion of people with disability. Disability policy includes:

- Strategies which typically centre on improving the lives of people with disability
- Guidelines which articulate the way in which disability policy should be enlivened
- Standards which specify minimum expectations of how services or goods should be provided in accordance with legislation, industry codes and conventions

Unlike other policy areas with well-established academic disciplines such as healthcare and education, disability policy is often considered a field within social sciences or law rather than a separate discipline in its own right (Staupe-Delgado et al., 2022; Lawson, 2020). This means that there may be a tendency for disability policymakers to draw heavily from other fields due to a lack of unified identity or a universally agreed upon specialist language (Staupe-Delgado et al., 2022; Lawson, 2020). Yet, researchers argue that it is crucially important for disability policy to be considered its own discipline in order to pay justice to and better understand the complex interplay of individual, social and systemic factors that impact the lives of people with disability (Lawson, 2020; Staupe-Delgado, 2022). A dedicated policy field allows for focused research, advocacy and policy codesign that directly addresses the needs and rights of the diverse population of people with disability. Further, the fact that people with disability make up the largest minority group on earth means that policies designed with their outcomes in mind should actively promote their inclusion, equal rights and participation in all aspects of life (Harte, 2025).

Common features of disability policy

Some common features of disability policy that have long been advocated for by people with disability, advocates and researchers include:

- Codesign: an approach which actively involves people with disability in the design and implementation of policies that affect them, placing their 'voice' at the centre of decision-making (Rieger, 2020).

- Intersectionality: a concept which recognises that disability doesn't exist in isolation. Rather, disability intersects with other aspects of a person's social identity. Race, gender, sexuality and socioeconomic status compound the barriers that people with disability face and result in new forms of discrimination (Brinkman, 2020).
- Lived experience: refers to the first-hand knowledge and insights gained by people with disability, and often their families/carers, about navigating daily life with disability (Boxall, 2018).
- Human rights-based approach: recognises people with disability as rights-holders, emphasising their autonomy and need for equal opportunity and participation in all aspects of life (Kayess, 2008).
- Social model of disability: This approach views disability as a social construct, resulting from societal barriers rather than individual 'impairments'. This approach places advocacy at its centre, promoting change in people's attitudes, behaviours and environments to advance inclusion (Barnes, 2001).

Features like codesign are increasingly recognised by policymakers as better practice in public policy settings. However, these features are not universally practiced among all policymakers (Fraser-Barbour et al., 2023). Furthermore, there may be significant variance in the way in which the aforementioned features are understood and applied in policy settings. In some cases, a lack of adherence to the principles and practices defined in the above features may result in policy that does not reflect the needs of people with disability and is therefore unlikely to achieve the intended outcomes. Codesign is a prime example of this, as it is often confused with feedback consultation. Within feedback-oriented consultation, relevant stakeholder views are sought but policy decisions are often made by others without consideration of the feedback received (JFA Purple Orange, 2021). In contrast to this form of consultation where stakeholders' feedback can be down-played or ignored entirely, codesign is a process whereby relevant stakeholder views contribute not only to the thinking behind decisions but also to making them (JFA Purple Orange, 2021). Feedback consultation tends to be used when policy decisions need to made quickly, whereas codesign tends to be embedded throughout the life course of research and policy development (JFA Purple Orange, 2021). When feedback consultation is misunderstood to be codesign, it dramatically limits policymakers' understanding of the problems being addressed, which can only be achieved by engaging meaningfully with stakeholders in a collaborative and iterative process (JFA Purple Orange, 2021). Furthermore, as feedback-oriented consultation focuses more on gathering comments on existing designs and proposals, those who mistake this form of consultation for codesign inadvertently limit their potential to be open to new ideas or approaches to addressing social problems (Malcolm, 2022). Consequently, 'good' codesign must be present at the start of the research and policy process, playing a critical role in informing decisions about what the problem is that needs to be solved and what appropriate solutions might look like, including levers for change.

Another contentious area known to trigger debate among policymakers pertains to evidence – what it is, what it is not and when and why it should be used. Most policymakers would agree that evidence plays a critical role in the development of 'good' disability policy. Evidence helps policymakers understand the nature, timing and extent of social problems and evaluate the potential effectiveness of different policy interventions. However, in public policy settings, 'evidence' usually pertains to a mix of political ideology, public opinion and consultation feedback (Cairney, 2016). In contrast, social policy researchers – who conduct research to inform social policy – often define evidence as rigorously tested, validated data and derived from quantitative and qualitative research (Head, 2008). In essence, public policymakers often prefer to draw from a wide range of anecdotal sources, and social policy researchers tend to be more 'purist' in their approach – believing that policy decisions should be based predominantly on empirical evidence and data analysis rather than public opinion or political ideology (Cairney, 2016; Head, 2008). Ideally, both approaches should be used to inform policy in order to increase the likelihood of it achieving its intended purpose. Knowledge of the political landscape and public opinion may help to ensure that policy is accepted and implemented in practice, and rigorously tested evidence can shape the content of policy to ensure that the 'right' things are considered in the 'right' way. One way in which policymakers are slowly starting to improve the rigour of the evidence they employ to inform their policy decisions is through implementation science.

Implementation science

Typically, implementation science is applied at the start of policy design, before work begins, to ensure that all the 'right things' are considered and thus the best outcomes achieved (Tabak, 2018). Questions are asked at the very beginning of the policy cycle with the 'big picture' in mind. 'Big picture' thinking provides insight into the necessary context for the task at hand. It allows one to understand how seemingly isolated policy work fits into a larger 'policy puzzle', including possible impacts, and any discrepancies that exist between the individual policy task and the wider context (Tabak, 2018). However, unlike traditional thinking that might focus on policy design or impact (e.g. will the policy achieve its intended outcome?), implementation science specifically examines the way in which processes, strategies and factors may influence how a policy is adopted, integrated, delivered and sustained in real-world settings (Tabak, 2018). For example, implementation science might ask how might this policy fail in practice? Other questions relevant to disability policy that a policymaker might ask through an implementation science lens include:

- What are the precise goals and objectives of this policy? Are they clear, measurable and relevant to the needs of people with disability?
- What underlying assumptions about disability, inclusion or support are being made relevant to the policy goal and objective?
- Does the policy clearly define the roles and responsibilities of different stakeholders (government agencies, service providers, individuals with disability, families)?
- Is the proposed policy topic (or its core components/interventions) truly evidence-based? What research supports its effectiveness in achieving desired outcomes for people with disability?
- Has the evidence been adapted or considered for the specific context of this policy (e.g. Australian context, specific types of disability, rural vs. urban)?
- What are the existing disability policies, legislation and funding models that this new policy interacts with? Are there potential overlaps, gaps or conflicts?

- What is the current political and social climate surrounding disability rights and inclusion? Is there strong political will and public support for the policy topic?
- How does the proposed policy align with broader national strategies (e.g. Australia's Disability Strategy 2021–2031) and international conventions (e.g. UNCRPD)?
- Which organisations, government departments and service providers will be responsible for implementing this policy? What are their current capacities, resources (financial, human, technological) and existing infrastructure?
- What is the organisational culture like within these implementing agencies? Is it open to change, collaborative, person-centred and inclusive of people with disability?
- Are there established interagency collaboration mechanisms? How well do different parts of the system communicate and co-ordinate?
- What knowledge, skills and attitudes do frontline staff (e.g. support workers, therapists, case managers, educators) need to effectively implement the policy? Do they currently possess these?
- What are the current workloads and pressures of frontline staff who would be responsible for implementing the policy? How might the policy impact their roles?
- What are the diverse needs, preferences and lived experiences of the people the policy is designed to help (e.g. people with various disabilities, their families and carers)?
- What are the potential barriers to access for different people with disability (e.g. geographic remoteness, cultural and linguistic diversity, digital exclusion)?
- How will people with disability and other relevant stakeholders be involved in evaluating the policy to ensure it has achieved its intended purpose?

Essentially, implementation science systematically identifies and categorises factors that hinder (barriers) or help (facilitators) policy realisation. Implementation science also recognises that successful policy implementation requires active involvement and collaboration among diverse stakeholders, including policymakers, government agencies, service providers, community organisations and the ultimate beneficiaries of the policy – people with disability.

Sense checking

Even when armed with answers to questions about policy goals and how the measures supporting them should be implemented, there remains another key practice that is often missed during the development of disability policy – sense checking. This step, typically initiated towards the end of a project, is about checking one's understanding of the policy problem and the proposed policy solutions (Head, 2008). In essence, sense checking is about asking people that the policy is designed to help, 'could this work'?; 'does it make sense'?; and 'have we considered all the right things'? Sense checking is a critical measure that can be employed early on in policy work to ensure that all relevant information has been considered and more importantly, interpreted correctly. It goes beyond engaging with stakeholders, which is typically used to inform thinking about a particular issue and how it can be solved. Sense checking involves checking if a policy solution is likely to work. It is an early attempt to rectify issues before they become problematic and costly.

People with lived experience of the contexts that policy is designed for are critical in the sense checking process. They know the existing barriers and enablers for policy implementation that already exist in these contexts and can inform decisions about whether or not policy solutions are likely to work. For disability policy, it is important to, first and foremost, include people with disability in 'sense checking' discussions. However, it is also very important to include the staff who support them, and also any other people who are significantly involved in their lives. Often, frontline staff who provide direct support to people with disability are not involved in discussions designed to inform policy; rather, management and senior leaders within organisations tend to be the people involved in these critical tasks (McEwen, 2022). Consequently, a valuable perspective is often lost that could provide a deep, firsthand knowledge about daily life in disability service contexts, which are frequently the focus of disability policy (McEwen, 2022). Frontline staff usually have an intimate understanding of the practical realities, challenges and successes experienced by people with disabilities in their everyday lives. They see how policies are played out in practice, and thus, often possess excellent knowledge about what does and does not work (McEwen, 2022).

Sense checking can also include piloting or testing a policy solution within the contexts it is designed for. Essentially, this approach allows policymakers to:

- Identify and mitigate unintended consequences
- Gather real-world feedback about what does and does not work
- Refine and optimise policy design
- Test feasibility and scalability
- Reduce risk before the cost of full implementation

Sense checking may also build trust and coalition between policymakers and those likely to be impacted by the policy; it may also build rapport and understanding among those responsible for its implementation. Essentially, sense checking provides an opportunity for policymakers and the intended recipients of policy to share information, test understanding and make clear policy intentions (Harkness & Benda, 2020). However, it is critical that sense checking is done reliably and authentically, otherwise the credibility of policymakers may be called into question (Cairney, 2016). Reliable, authentic sense checking can be achieved by policymakers assigning adequate time for the process, limiting the need to rush and apply pressure to those involved. Avoiding rushed timelines for sense checking policy knowledge and proposed policy solutions are especially important for people with disability, who may require additional time to engage meaningfully in the process (Fraser-Barbour et al., 2023). This is particularly important for individuals with 'less visible' forms of disability, including those who identify as neurodivergent. Policymakers should also ensure they check with stakeholders about what they need to engage meaningfully in the sense checking process, as they may require resources or adjustments, including:

- Information and time ahead of meetings
- Time during meetings to process questions and clarify meaning before responding
- A clear order of communication for meetings to ensure they have equal opportunity to contribute

Building coalition

Stakeholder analysis is often where engagement with the individuals who are likely to be impacted by policy begins and ends. However, for policymakers who genuinely want to see their policy goals realised, one needs to move beyond engagement and towards 'building coalition'. Building coalition involves policymakers taking stakeholders 'along the policy journey' with them (Ansell & Gash, 2008). It's about engaging often to share information and to create an authentic dialogue rather than engagement being centred around specific feedback points in the policy lifecycle. Policymakers need not wait until they have something significant to share before they engage with stakeholders. By sharing information little and often, policymakers allow people to see them as transparent and collaborative, and there are no surprises when policy is finally released. This approach may forge trust and save time when policy is disseminated, as key groups of individuals will already be aware of its content and will therefore be less likely to contest it.

Separating the part from the whole

Sometimes, public policy problems are approached in isolation, without considering the full context of issues that intersect with and compound the problem the policy is attempting to solve (Cairney, 2016). However, in public policy, the problems that policymakers want to solve are deeply intertwined with broader social, economic, cultural and political issues. For example, poverty, often experienced by people with disability around the world, is frequently linked to unemployment, poor health, lack of education and housing insecurity. Further, mental health issues can be exacerbated by social isolation, financial stress or discrimination. Addressing one part of a public policy problem without considering its interconnectedness with other parts can result in policy failing to address its intended outcomes (Cairney, 2016). This may result in misconceptions that the policy problem at hand is not solvable or that the policy levers prescribed to address it do not work.

It is also important to consider that people with disability, like all people, need to be viewed holistically – they too have complex lives, relationships and needs (Fraser-Barbour et al., 2023). Disability is only one part of a person's identity. Therefore, by focusing on just one aspect of a person's identity, such as job readiness through the provision of, for example, training, without addressing other barriers to employment, such as a lack of available childcare or transportation, policy solutions are unlikely to prove successful.

Knowledge mobilisation

Ensuring that a policy is 'mobilised', that is, it is realised in practice, can be challenging. Even when a policymaker considers implementation, sense checks policy approaches with key stakeholders and ensures that the policy is progressed in the context of other interconnected social issues, it can still fail to be realised in practice. Consequently, policymakers must consider how they intend to 'mobilise' policy, a task which is heavily reliant on drawing on relationships fostered through coalition building activities, to ensure that policy is widely understood. In the context of disability policy, being 'widely understood' is heavily dependent on the way in which information is presented and disseminated. Information should be 'in Plain Language', avoiding jargon, acronyms and overly complex sentence structures (Harpur & O'Toole, 2022). However, Plain Language is not just useful for people with cognitive or intellectual disability, it is also important for anyone who will be responsible for enlivening policy in some way. Evidence suggests that approximately 44% of Australian adults (aged 15–74) have low or very low literacy skills (Australian Bureau of Statistics, 2013). Further, approximately 22.3% of Australians speak a language other than English at home (Australian Bureau of Statistics, 2022). Therefore, one could argue that Plain Language policy is not only beneficial for people with cognitive or intellectual disability, but for everyone.

Guidance material can also be useful in mobilising policy knowledge. However, traditional guidance material, like policy, is in written formats. It may be useful for policymakers to consider other modes of guidance that are more accessible for a wider variety of individuals. For example, guidance can be provided in video format, podcast or even within interactive platforms that combine these modes of communication in a variety of language options. However, it is important to remember that not everyone has high levels of digital literacy, and therefore, it is critical to keep information as simple and accessible as possible (Harkness & Benda, 2020). Testing information in a variety of formats and with a wide variety of people is a good way to tease out any issues with the accessibility of content before disseminating policy and any associated guidance material.

Evaluation

Evaluation is key to ensuring that policy is achieving its intended outcomes (Cairney, 2016). Without evaluation, there is a risk that policy will be considered as achieving its intended purpose or 'working', when it may not be. Even when policy appears to be yielding positive results, there are always lessons that can be shared about how future policy can improve. Further, evaluation may shed light on positive practice for policy design and implementation that should be tracked for replication (Head, 2008). In essence, by investing in evaluation, policymakers learn about what did and did not work during the policy design process and what is and is not working in practice. However, evaluation is often missing from policymaking, resulting in many questions about implementation and outcomes left unanswered (Cairney, 2016; Head, 2008).

In the context of Australian disability policy, few evaluations have been conducted over time; hence, little is known about their impacts on the lives of people with disability. This is largely because data on issues such as disability education and employment can be complex and sometimes confusing due to various factors, including the diversity of people's disabilities, differences in reporting methodologies and challenges in accessing and analysing data. Consequently, evaluation that focuses on the lived experience of people with disability is of critical importance, as it allows for a deeper exploration of issues which are enabling or disabling people with disabilities from living a 'good' life (Rieger, 2020). These insights allow policymakers to make inferences about the impacts of policy, and the factors which may or may not be working and in what contexts.

Conclusion

Ultimately, the path towards effective disability policy rests not in one single act, but a continuous, adaptive and human-centred process. It begins by elevating the centrality of lived experience and recognising it as the foundational knowledge that informs every stage. Qualitative expertise is then systematically integrated through genuine codesign and rigorous sense checking, ensuring that solutions are not only theoretically sound but also practical and aligned with the real needs of people with disability. Successful policy is also a collective effort, requiring broad coalition building to achieve a holistic vision that deliberately aims to move beyond fragmented support to create integrated, person centred systems. Finally, the sustainability of these efforts depends on a robust cycle of learning – leveraging implementation science to translate policy into practice, engaging in active knowledge mobilisation to share what works and building a strong framework for evaluation to measure real-world impact and drive ongoing improvement. This comprehensive approach transforms policy from a static document into a dynamic tool for fostering empowerment, inclusion and equity.

References

Ansell, C., & Gash, A. (2008). Collaborative Governance in Theory and Practice. *Journal of Public Administration Research and Theory, 18*(4), 543–571.

Australian Bureau of Statistics (ABS). (2022). *2021 Census: Cultural diversity data summary*. Cat. No. 2071.0.

Australian Bureau of Statistics. (2013). *Programme for the International Assessment of Adult Competencies, Australia, 2011–2012*. Cat. No. 4228.0.

Barnes, C., & Mercer, G. (Eds.). (2001). *Disability: The Social Model of Disability*. Polity Press.

Boxall, K., Johnson, A., Mitting, L., Simpson, S., Zwickl, S., & Zwickl, J. (2018). Disability policy and lived experience: reflections from regional Australia. In P. Beresford & S. Carr (Eds.), *Social policy first hand: an international introduction to participatory social welfare.* Policy Press.

Brinkman, A., Rea-Sandin, G., Lund, E., Fitzpatrick, O., Gusman, M., & Boness, C. (2020). Shifting the discourse on disability: Moving to an inclusive, intersectional focus. *American Journal of Orthopsychiatry* 2023;93(1):50–62. doi: 10.1037/ort0000653.

Cairney, P. (2016). *The Politics of Evidence-Based Policy Making.* Palgrave Macmillan.

Fraser-Barbour, E., Robinson, S., Gendera, S., Burton-Clark, I., Fisher, K. R., Alexander, J., & Howe, K. (2023). Shifting power to people with disability in co-designed research. *Disability & Society, 40*(2), 1–22.

Harkness, S., & Benda, J. (2020). Designing for implementation: A new approach to policy making. *Journal of Policy Practice, 19*(2), 171–188

Harpur, A., & O'Toole, L. (2022). Implementing a Human Rights Framework for Disability: What Does It Mean for a Service Provider?. *Journal of Law and Society, 49*(3), 392–411.

Harte, B. (2025). How intersectionality impacts people with a disability –and what we can do about it. Retrieved from: https://missingperspectives.com/posts/intersectionality-disability/

Head, B. W. (2008). Three Lenses of Evidence-Based Policy. *Australian Journal of Public Administration, 67*(1), 1–11.

JFA Purple Orange. (2021). *Guide to Co-Design with People living with disability.* Retrieved from: https://purpleorange.org.au/what-we-do/library-our-work/guide-co-design-people-living-disability.

Kayess, R., & French, P. (2008). Out of Darkness into Light? The Case of the Convention on the Rights of Persons with Disabilities. *Human Rights Law Review, 8*(1), 1–33.

Lawson, A. (2020). Disability Law as an Academic Discipline: Towards Cohesion and Mainstreaming?. *Journal of Law and Society, 47*(4), 558–587.

Malcolm, J. (2022). *The Impact of Co-design on Policy Outcomes in the Social Services Sector*. The Social Policy Review, 15(2), 45–62.

McEwen, Jade (2022). Regulatory Ritualism Exploring Australian Governments' Approach to Monitoring Quality in Disability Services. La Trobe. Thesis. https://doi.org/10.26181/21386247.v1

Rieger, J. (2020). *Right to Participate: Co-designing Disability Policies in Australia*. QUT Centre for Justice Briefing Papers, 12, pp. 1–4. Retrieved from: https://research.qut.edu.au/centre-for-justice/wp-content/uploads/sites/304/2021/02/Briefing-paper-series-Dec-2020-Issue12.pdf.

Staupe-Delgado, R. (2022). *Disability and public policy: A scoping review of the literature*. Norwegian Centre for Human Rights, University of Oslo.

Tabak, R. G., Padek, M. M., & Brownson, R. C. (2018). The Evolution of Implementation Science. *Frontiers in Public Health, 6*, 223

3

Seeing the person before the problem: Using lived experience perspectives to eliminate restrictive practices

Bethany Easton, Kyle Moat, Edward Creamer, Ebony Mychajlyk and Niall Hewitt

Introduction

We begin our chapter by introducing a case study about Henry and his lived experience of disability and restrictive practices.

Henry is happiest sitting under a tree, touching the earth, leaves and long grass that he finds there. Aged in his early 30s, Henry has been living in supported accommodation since he was 14. He is autistic, and lives with an intellectual disability and anxiety. He doesn't speak, and has a history of using physical behaviour towards others to communicate his wants and needs.

Since his early 20s, Henry has lived by himself with 24-hour supports, assisted by two staff members at all waking hours. An assault towards a staff member when Henry was 24 years old resulted in him becoming subject to significant restrictions. His community access was limited to being taken by staff for walks in the park and to a local pool. However, after he behaved aggressively towards other people during one of these outings, Henry's accommodation provider completed a workplace health and safety assessment, which determined that the risk of taking him into the community was too high. Henry's access to the community then ceased. Apart from daily car rides during which he was secured by a harness into his seat, Henry did not leave his home for more than 5 years.

Henry's home was also heavily restricted. Large parts of the home included safety glass screens to create a barrier for staff; he had only intermittent contact with support workers, occasional contact with his family and no contact with anyone else. Henry was not included in the decision-making about the restrictions that were imposed on him.

Henry's experience may be extreme, but it is unfortunately not unique. Across the globe, people with disabilities are frequently subject to restrictive and coercive practices (Bartlett & Ellis, 2020; Fitton & Jones, 2020; Younan et al., 2024). Restrictive practices refer to physical, pharmacological, environmental, mechanical, seclusive or other punitive methods used to limit a person's freedom of movement in response to behaviours that are deemed a problem by the people who support them (often called 'challenging behaviours'). Restrictive practices occur in disability services, schools, prisons, aged and healthcare settings as well as family homes. Safety concerns for the person with a disability or those around them are a common justification for their use (Spivakovsky et al., 2023). And yet, restrictive practices have been shown to be stressful and painful for people with disabilities, who often have limited understanding of when or why they are to be used (Griffith et al., 2013).

There is, however, a broad policy imperative for change. The UNCRPD (2006) prohibits its 164 member states from discrimination on the basis of disability and affirms the inherent dignity and autonomy of all people with disability. The active efforts of UN Special Rapporteurs to scrutinise restrictive practices sit alongside increasing public awareness of their harmful use (see, e.g., Aguilar & Pūras, 2015; BBC, 2022; CNN, 2011; Connolly, 2023). Governments, health, education and community service authorities in countries, including Australia, Indonesia, Ireland, the United Kingdom, the United States, New Zealand, Sweden and the Netherlands, are exploring or have endorsed policy positions to reduce or eliminate the use of restrictive practices towards people with disabilities.

Despite evidence of the inherent risks of restrictive practices, policies to reduce or eliminate their use remain mostly unrealised. The perspectives of people with disabilities who are subject to restrictions are scant in research and policymaking. Where lived experience accounts do exist, people who have experienced restrictive practices emphasise both unintended consequences and preferable alternative approaches, and this has important implications for policy and practice. In this chapter, we begin by reporting on a pressing policy issue, being the lack of lived experience research used to inform current restrictive practice policy in Australia and around the world. Following on, we identify barriers and enablers to participating in restrictive practice-related disability research and policy development for people with disabilities, in particular autistic people, people with an intellectual disability and people with complex communication needs. We then extend our critical discussion about restrictive practice research and policy inclusion to cover children and young people with disabilities. Finally, we draw on our experience as practitioner-researchers to outline the need and potential scope for a lived experience research agenda that reflects the diverse profile and stories of people with disabilities who are subjected to restrictive interventions. Such an agenda will help illuminate the human costs and person-centred solutions that hold promise for the reduction or elimination of restrictive practices.

The policy issue – Few lived experience perspectives inform restrictive practice policy

From where we write in Australia, very little research draws on the experiences of people with disabilities who have been subject to restrictive practices. Instead, participatory research relating to restrictive practices tends to focus on mental health inpatient settings and the use of physical restraint, mechanical restraint and seclusion (Brophy et al., 2016; Cortis et al., 2023). Studies over the past 30 years have illuminated the human impact of restrictive practices in mental healthcare, a toll that includes emotional distress, trauma and re-traumatisation, isolation, feelings of dehumanisation and a markedly diminished sense of self (Meehan et al., 2000; Roper et al., 2021). People subject to restrictive practices in Australian mental health settings are more likely to view the practices as harmful than the professionals who implement them (Kinner et al., 2017), and it has been argued that the professional lexicon surrounding restrictive practices serves to sanitise and legitimate them (Brophy et al., 2016). Consequently, it is no surprise that a recent inquiry into the mental health system in the south-eastern state of Victoria (State of Victoria, 2021) stressed the importance of programmes being codesigned between mental health services and the people they serve, in an effort to end within the next decade the use of seclusion and restraint in the sector.

Of the lived experience research into restrictive practices that has occurred to Australians with disabilities, findings echo those from the mental health sector. As part of the national Royal Commission into Violence, Abuse, Neglect and Exploitation of People with Disability (2023), submissions and private hearings enabled people who had been subject to restrictive practices to share their experiences. One participant explained that her experience of chemical restraint and seclusion in a hospital psychiatric ward 'deeply added to the trauma [she] was already suffering' (Commonwealth of Australia, 2023, p.523). Another who had been subject to chemical restraint in a youth justice setting said that he simply 'didn't want to see others go through this' (Commonwealth of Australia, 2023, p. 435). In research requested by the Royal Commission, Spivakovsky et al. (2023) reviewed existing lived experience research from people with disabilities who had been subject to restrictive practices, highlighting the presence of trauma, abandonment, fear and unequal power dynamics within care relationships where restrictive practices are present. The Royal Commission into Violence, Abuse, Neglect and Exploitation of People with Disability (Commonwealth of Australia, 2023) demonstrated that the perspectives of people with disabilities who have been subjected to restrictive practices stand in contrast to contemporary Australian frameworks for supporting people with disabilities who use challenging behaviours, including frontline behavioural interventions such as positive behaviour support, which have arguably shifted the emphasis towards documenting and authorising restrictive interventions rather than reducing them (Hayward et al., 2022). Promisingly, the current Australian federal government has recently pledged extensive resources towards actioning the recommendations outlined in the report, which includes AUD 1.2 million to develop targets to reduce and eliminate restrictive practices (Ministers for the Department of Social Services, 2024

Internationally, the picture is similar. The voices of people with lived experience of restrictive practices are most evident in research related to mental health inpatient settings (Franks et al., 2021). Mental healthcare has seen an international movement towards embedding lived experience in policymaking, service design and delivery, thereby 'harnessing the expertise of experience' (Perkins et al., 2010, p.13). Even so, an international scoping review of 121 English-language studies related to preventing and reducing coercive practices in mental health services found few studies that had involved people who had received mental health services or been subject to involuntary interventions, either as participants or as researchers (Gooding et al., 2020).

The limited studies highlighting perspectives of people with disabilities who have been involved in decision-making related to restrictive practices hold important insights for policy and practice. For example, a synthesis of perspectives of people with intellectual disabilities and challenging behaviours (Griffith et al., 2013) showed that feeling disrespected and disempowered in residential services tends to precipitate challenging behaviours, which, in turn, leads to residents being further harmed through the use of restrictive practices. A study from Norway (Røstad et al., 2023) reviewed the restrictive practice authorisation documents for 120 people with intellectual disabilities and found that restrictive practices reduced year on year when participants were involved in describing their own life situation and empowered to make decisions relating to their care. This pattern was repeated where disability services understood the triggers of a person's challenging behaviour and had access to an individualised support plan. These lived experience perspectives contrast starkly with responses from Swedish staff asked to consider organisational changes required to prevent restrictive practice in day services and group homes (Björne et al., 2022), in which respondents overwhelmingly identified structural changes like environmental modifications, additional staffing, training and supervision rather than resident-centred approaches, although some staff did note that low arousal alternatives could prevent the need for restrictive practices.

It is evident that opinions about the risks, benefits and viable alternatives to restrictive practices differ between people who have been subject to restrictive practices and the professionals responsible for implementing them. The current lack of lived experience perspectives in restrictive practice research therefore obstructs attempts to understand the diverse and complex experiences of people with disabilities across a variety of settings (Giri et al., 2022). This is despite the lived experience research to date indicating that the needs and priorities of the disability community cannot be met through policy or practice without centring the subjective experiences of people with disabilities (Ferguson & Nusbaum, 2012). It is perhaps for this reason that the UN Secretary General António Guterres has underscored the need for people with disabilities to be 'fully included in decision-making processes on all issues that affect them' (United Nations, 2023) lest progress on disability inclusion begin a backward slide.

There are some encouraging Australian and international initiatives that have involved people with disabilities in developing policy practice resources to reduce restrictive practices. In the United Kingdom, the *Restraint Reduction Network Training Standards* (Ridley & Leitch, 2021) were developed with the involvement of people who have experienced restraint. All mental health, learning disability and autism services funded by the UK National Health Service must be certified against these standards. *Deciding with Support* (Flinders University & Council for Intellectual Disability, n.d.) is a suite of accessible resources, codesigned with people with disabilities. The resources are intended to facilitate involving people with disabilities who demonstrate challenging behaviours as their own behaviour support plans are developed. While promising, these initiatives have yet to be evaluated for their efficacy in reducing restrictive practices. The State of Victoria is currently developing a strategy towards the elimination of seclusion and restraint in mental health services, using a codesign process with people who have experienced or felt at risk of experiencing restrictive practices (Department of Health, 2023); however, as noted, this strategy is still in development.

Whether in Australia or abroad, many other policy initiatives to reduce restrictive practices conspicuously lack the involvement of people who have experienced restrictive practices in their design, delivery and evaluation (Spivakovsky et al., 2023). Given the persistence of restrictive practices towards people with disability, the significant harms associated with their use and the fundamental need to include people with disabilities in all decisions that affect them, there is a clear imperative for lived experience perspectives to better inform restrictive practice policy. Below, we outline further considerations to address disability research and policy participation challenges for three groups of people with disability who are vulnerable to restrictive practices: autistic people; people with intellectual disabilities or complex communication needs; and children.

Restrictive practice-related disability research and policy – Participation barriers and enablers for autistic people, people with an intellectual disability and people with complex communication needs

There has been a growth in self-report methods for research with autistic people, indicating that this is increasingly being recognised as the most appropriate and efficacious methodology to meaningfully engage and enact positive change with this cohort (Huang et al., 2020). There is a clear need for research to be conducted with rather than about autistic people (Jones et al., 2021). Generally speaking, research involving autistic people often focuses on parents' perspectives and opinions regarding their autistic children (Anderberg & South, 2021; Downes et al., 2020; Jacobs et al., 2020; Poslawsky et al., 2014; Rasmussen et al., 2020; Reed & Osborne, 2019). However, there is a notable scarcity of similar research for autistic adults; research on autistic adults is significantly under-represented when compared to the volume of research on autistic children (Damiano et al., 2014). Further, there is a bias of gender in the samples of many contemporary studies, where most studies of autistic adults involve a male-majority sample (Huang et al., 2020).

A common co-existing condition with autism is intellectual disability (Matson & Shoemaker, 2009); however, research samples involving participants with both diagnoses is lacking. While research does include people with intellectual disability, there are very few randomised controlled trials that are considered the 'gold standard' of evidence, which involves those with intellectual disability (Lennox et al., 2005). Lennox et al. (2005) described barriers to involving people with intellectual disabilities in disability research (encompassing research about restrictive practices), which include:

- Organisational barriers: 'Top heavy' organisations in which there are many levels of management between the nominated liaison person for the project and the potential participant with the disability, leading to inertia or blocked communication.

- Accessibility barriers: In Australia, there is no accessible register of adults with intellectual disability that can be recruited for intervention studies, making it difficult to identify and access populations to perform these studies. Additionally, some individuals may be living independently of formal supports, may have a lack of access to their community due to their disability needs or may be unknown to service organisations.
- Funding constraints: Individuals with intellectual disability and the people who support them may receive inadequate funding, contributing to a lack of connection with services that could be used for the recruitment process.
- Demands of caring: Those who care for people with intellectual disability may not have the capacity to undertake or facilitate participation in research. The study references a parent who stated that they would have liked to participate in the study as a carer, but simply did not have the energy to do so, viewing the study participation as an optional additional load which became a low priority.
- Consent issues: Many adults with intellectual disability cannot consent to participation themselves, often requiring substituted decision-making; a third party is needed to give consent on their behalf, elongating the length of the recruitment process.
- Perception of the word 'advocacy': Researchers described a problem with families being unfamiliar with the term, resulting in a hesitancy to be involved in research.
- Discrimination: People with intellectual disabilities and their support network may be distrustful of 'specialists' due to perceived negative experiences when they were supported in the past. The study did not elaborate on what these

experiences were; however, this could possibly include feeling misunderstood, dismissed or not listened to.

- Ethics: Ethical limitations prevent direct recruitment of potential participants. While this safeguard is necessary to protect those with disabilities, it may also have an impact of reducing the inclusion of the person with disability or their carers in disability research.

Additionally, a scoping review of the intellectual disability literature for 2001–2015 conducted by Dean et al. (2016) identified the problem of intellectual disability research not having a consistent definition of what 'participation' means for this population, despite having good intentions of focussing on the outcome of including more people with intellectual disability. The researchers argued that this results in certain domains of lived experience, such as choice and responsibility, not being adequately represented in participation literature. This is an important consideration as the more consistent the literature is, the easier a consensus can be reached around the definition of participation, which can then help to inform and support approaches and policy changes involving restrictive practices that are relevant to the people with disabilities themselves.

Not using verbal language and having a severe or profound intellectual disability can severely restrict a person's ability to communicate their experiences, even with the best supports provided. It is often those supporting the person with disability who must interpret and relay the experience, and in our experience when working with families and services, it is often these same people who are implementing the restrictive practices. Further, challenging behaviours are often adaptations to difficult environments. It is important to recognise the impact that communal-supported accommodation settings have in producing behaviours (Ramcharan et al., 2009), and how restrictive practices can be maintained by the environment, systems and supports the person with disability lives within.

As disability practitioners, we have seen that for people with intellectual disability and complex communication needs, even with the best intentions, the capacity and resources of a person's supporters can often be a major barrier to reducing restrictive practices. The advent or increase in restrictive practices is often a risk management strategy to a challenging behaviour, coupled with deficits in resources, training, confidence, skills and knowledge within the person's support system (Carter, 2006). This can contribute to and ultimately embed restrictive practices that often continue to be enacted even when there is no evidence that they are still required for an individual. A family's capacity, staff attitudes, organisational culture, fear, occupational health and safety and systemic barriers, including funding limitations, all may be factors that limit opportunities for successful implementation of 'fade out plans'. If you have an intellectual disability and live in accommodation and support settings, the timeline for restrictive practice reduction is often set based on the supporters and service management being willing and able to implement change, which may be slow to establish or never happen. Both professional staff and residents of long-term care for people with intellectual disability seek stability and predictability (Bisschops et al., 2022). Authorisation and oversight are often insufficient to assure rights to liberty and security on an equal basis of a person with disability, particularly intellectual or cognitive disability

(McSherry & Maker, 2021). Richardson et al. (2019) found that restrictive practices remained for at least 3 years for people with intellectual disability or developmental delay in Australia.

For example, Giuseppe who has a severe intellectual disability, is autistic and does not use verbal language. As a child, he experienced significant trauma and entered an institution for the intellectually disabled in the 1980s in Australia. As a likely self-protective behaviour and to express his distress, he used aggressive behaviour towards others and self-harm through banging his head. Over many years, he was prescribed an increasing level of chemical restraint medication, which further decreased his ability to effectively communicate and engage with others. Giuseppe's use of challenging behaviour to have his needs met, the inability of support staff to interpret the meaning of his communication efforts and a lack of understanding of the personal impact of restraint medication prescribed led to increases in medication throughout his 20s and 30s until Giuseppe was taking over forty individual tablets per day. After many years, the side effects from the prescribed medication cocktail brought about a painful underlying issue, although this remained undetected for some time. The condition seemed to induce Giuseppe to hit himself hard on the chest and increasingly bang his head. His actions continued to be viewed by his support service and treating doctor through the lens of challenging behaviour related to his disability, not the communication of his pain and expression of his experience. Consequently, his chemical restraint medication was increased, and a very painful gastrointestinal condition went undiagnosed and untreated for many years.

The question for researchers, policymakers, disability providers and supports should be: is the challenging behaviour of a person who does not use verbal language effectively (or is not being effectively supported by their communication partner/ support worker) the voice that is communicating pain, dissatisfaction, protest and resistance? The very fact that behaviours of protest are occurring indicates that the rights of the person are not being upheld and their experience of their situation is not being heard. Amplifying their voice, listening and understanding the impact of restrictive practices must underpin the efforts to reduce or eliminate the practice of restricting the human rights of this vulnerable population.

Restrictive practice-related disability research and policy – Participation barriers and enablers for children and young people with disabilities

Arya is 10 years old. She loves learning about the solar system and singing along to the 1980s rock ballads. She lives with her parents and younger siblings. She is autistic and lives with ADHD (attention-deficit/hyperactivity disorder) and anxiety. She has been supported by a team of medical and allied health professionals since toddlerhood. Arya manages her anxiety with predictability. Knowing what to expect each day, and making choices about where, how and with whom she spends her time, help Arya to feel calm and in control. School can be a challenging place for Arya – it's hard to make friends and she often has meltdowns when she gets home at the end of the day. Rigid rules, group activities, substitute teachers and timetable changes feel completely overwhelming. When Arya is very upset, she finds it hard to access her normal speech. Instead, she might use a few gestures or ignore the people around her. At times, she says offensive things or walks away from other people just to be left alone. Recently, Arya swore at a teacher who was telling her off in front of the class. The teacher began to cry, and so Arya was sent home. Later that day and in the weeks following, Arya talked a lot about wanting to hurt herself and wanting to disappear. She saw her psychologist and paediatrician, who recommended an atypical antipsychotic to reduce Arya's distress and prevent further agitation. After seeking a second opinion, Arya and her parents agreed to give it a go. Since starting the medication, Arya has felt a lot better, and the school staff seem pleased too. Arya's parents feel relieved and worried about the medication; the local authorising body considers it a chemical restraint because it was prescribed primarily to influence Arya's behaviour, and she is deemed to be too young to provide informed consent.

Children and young people with disabilities are particularly vulnerable to the physical, social and psychological harm posed by restrictive practices. For children, being subject to restrictive practices may intersect with experiences of trauma (Baker et al., 2022), abandonment or neglect (Spivakovsky et al., 2023), abuse or bullying (Children and Young People with Disability Australia [CYDA], 2016) and discrimination (Poed et al., 2020). The use of restrictive practices with children not only undermines therapeutic relationships and interventions (Baker et al., 2022; Willis et al., 2021), but can also be catastrophic. For example, between 1993 and 2018, restraint contributed to the deaths of seventy-nine children and adolescents in disability, mental health, correctional and out-of-home care settings across the United States (Nunno et al., 2022).

While the prevalence of restrictive interventions used with children is difficult to ascertain (Baker et al., 2022), it is evident that children with disabilities may experience these practices in schools, accommodation and youth justice settings, health and community services and in the family home. These restrictions could look like being secluded at school or placed on a restricted timetable as a behaviour management strategy: locked doors, windows and pantries in residential settings that exceed reasonable child safety precautions, or the prescription of medication to sedate the child or suppress menstruation due to behavioural concerns.

There have been few documented efforts to include children in research or policymaking related to restrictive practices, although some small samples exist (see, e.g., Willis et al., 2021). There are several barriers to the meaningful involvement of children with disabilities in these activities, including:

- The additional time and cost associated with facilitating ethical research with or supporting the involvement of children with disabilities, especially in relation to potentially harmful experiences.
- Children's learnt acceptance or normalisation of restrictive practices that occur within caregiving relationships or familiar settings (see Spivakovsky et al., 2023, pp.189–90).
- Expressive language or other communication difficulties that can make it difficult to convey the detail of their experiences or perspectives.

- Their ability to understand and provide consent due to their age and cognitive capacity.

More often, parents participate in research and advocacy efforts, speaking on behalf of their child's experiences. In Australia, parents of children with disability have spoken of how difficult it is to access information relating to restrictive practices used in schools or how their children's access to services was at times contingent on the use of restrictive practices (CYDA, 2016; Spivakovsky et al., 2023). Children and their parents have reflected that often, an upsetting interaction with a peer or caregiving adult or being forced into an uncomfortable environment is the trigger for the child's challenging behaviour, which they used as a means of communicating distress or protest. This, in turn, prompts a restrictive intervention which the child also experiences as aversive (Spivakovsky et al., 2023; Willis et al., 2021). Parents offer invaluable insight into children's experiences of restrictive practices. However, the stigma they experience in association with their child's behaviour (McLean & Halstead, 2021), well-founded fears about trialling less restrictive alternatives (Leif et al., 2023) and comparatively high rates of parental stress (Ashworth et al., 2019) are also likely to make it more difficult for parents of children with disabilities to engage in research and advocacy efforts.

Participatory research relating to children's experiences of restrictive practices is needed to illuminate the current scope of these practices as well as the approaches that can better protect children in different settings. Given indications that children's use of challenging behaviours is often a response to aversive interactions and environments, describing these experiences and evaluating children's preferred alternatives are important lines of enquiry.

The meaningful participation of children with disabilities in restrictive practice research and policymaking initiatives will require dedicated efforts from researchers. Useful strategies identified through a systemic review of research involving children and young people with disabilities (Bailey et al., 2015) include: making extra time and resourcing available to undertake research and engagement activities; ensuring supporting materials are accessible and provided in multiple formats; using flexible and engaging research activities; and remaining sensitive to the balance of power.

Given the particular vulnerability of children with disabilities to the harms of restrictive practices, it is important to underscore the need to attend to power dynamics inherent in research and policymaking processes. Activities seeking to engage children with disabilities who have been subject to restrictive practices should be separated from the services upon which the child or their family relies, offer children choices about how to engage on each occasion, ensure the availability of a trusted support person, ensure the timing and setting of each activity is convenient and comfortable for the child and their caregiver and make specialist debriefing and support accessible as required.

Co-designed research challenges and opportunities to eliminate or reduce restrictive practices – A lived experience research agenda

A good starting point for including people with disability in restrictive practice policy development is to have more accurate insights into the scope of their experiences. While inexact definitions and data lacking detail hinder policymakers' ability to gain clarity, lived experience accounts and information on best practice interventions could elucidate some significant considerations.

Many jurisdictions and service systems routinely collect data about restrictive practices to monitor, authorise and review their use. However, this data is not always made publicly available, and the lack of consistent operational definitions across jurisdictions means that data collation and comparison are compromised (Commonwealth of Australia, 2023; Fitton & Jones, 2020; Younan et al., 2024). Quantifying restrictive practice use is further complicated by poor agreement between professionals as to which practices are restrictive and unreliable documentation of their use (Schippers et al., 2018). These factors undermine efforts to develop cohesive policy frameworks for the monitoring and authorisation of restrictive practices (Hui et al., 2016).

We propose that meaningful participation of people with disabilities in codesigned studies about restrictive practices is a priority to informing related evidence-based policies. Current research shows us that not all disability studies are focussed on the benefits that those with lived experience of disability value, which can negatively impact participation rates. Future studies should focus on these values when undergoing recruitment of participants with disabilities. McDonald et al. (2016) demonstrated that those with intellectual disabilities value participation in a study when the benefits are framed altruistically, such as helping others and educating the community on disability, as well as mentioning direct benefits for the individual, such as learning new things, meeting new people, doing something new and receiving incentives. While these findings are helpful for improving participation in those with intellectual disabilities, similar research should be conducted on other groups, especially those with co-occurring conditions often left out of disability research studies. Anecdotally, many of the people we work with have multiple disabilities, whose voices are necessary if we are to have a meaningful policy change concerning restrictive practices. Additionally, given the bias of research samples towards certain genders (e.g. autism research has tended to include male participants), participation drives or opportunities for consultation would need to be gender-specific to allow for a broader voice and to correct for existing biases.

Further, when evaluating this research base with people with intellectual disability, there is a notable gap in the samples studied when considering the level of intellectual disability. Most research involves participants with a mild or moderate intellectual disability – often, research samples lack inclusion of those with severe or profound intellectual disabilities and often lacks those with complex communication needs. More research participation, and consequently codesign of policy, is required with this group; however, it is noted that this would be a challenging endeavour that would require careful ethical consideration. People with complex communication needs, who may be non-verbal or minimally verbal, often rely on their carers to interpret their perspectives, needs and wants when communicating with others. While including a trusted support person who is familiar with the person's communication style in the research process would increase participation rates, it also raises ethical concerns as the support person may be involved in the implementation of restrictive practices, which could lead to a confounding effect on the research outcomes.

A potential solution to this problem could be the development of a standardised method of generating a personalised communication strategy when supporting the participation of those with severe or profound intellectual disabilities and complex communication needs in research studies. Such an approach could include consultation with the person's wider support network as well as independent observation of the person in their common environments to determine their idiosyncratic communication needs. Researchers would also have to demonstrate flexibility; as this is such a varied cohort, research methodology would have to be malleable enough to allow for varied styles of communication.

A common shortfall in existing disability research is to sample populations with a single diagnosis (Hughes, 2023). In restrictive practice research, little evidence exists about how women, children, Aboriginal people and people from LGBTQIA+ (lesbian, gay, bisexual, transgender, queer/questioning, intersex, and asexual, with the plus sign acknowledging other identities) and culturally diverse communities experience restrictive interventions (Cortis et al., 2023; Roper et al., 2021). Without this, it is not possible to undertake intersectional analysis of multiple dimensions of identity as they relate to experiences of restrictive practices. Rather than recording individual instances of restraint and seclusion performed at a service level, a more holistic profile of restrictive practices should be built around the people subject to them, and would include:

- Demographic and personal characteristics, including age, locale, gender, sexual and cultural identity, income and education status.
- Disability details, including communication preferences, diagnoses and functional capacity.
- Types of restrictive practices experienced on a routine or ad hoc basis as well as the setting, frequency and duration.
- Whether the restrictive practice was used in accordance with an individualised support plan and whether the person with disability was involved in the development of that plan.

To take a meaningful and comprehensive view of restrictive practices, it is critical that the above data takes account of the multiple service systems used by people with disabilities. People who are subject to restrictive practices may experience forms of restraint in many parts of their lives, including in their home, in health and community services and at their school or day programmes. To capture this information would require high-level co-ordination across sectors and jurisdictions or the inclusion of restrictive practice questions in large-scale representative surveys. For example, the World Health Organisation and World Bank's *Model Disability Survey* (2017), which asked people with disabilities about their experience of being respected in healthcare settings and involved in treatment decisions, failed to capture information about experiences of restrictive practices.

Being able to reliably document and describe experiences of restrictive practices from the viewpoint of people with disability would illuminate groups who are more vulnerable to certain types of restrictive practices over longer periods or across multiple settings. Disaggregated data could show how restrictive practice use differs by sectors and regions, which is necessary to reliably target and evaluate policy interventions to reduce and remove restrictive practices.

Of course, descriptive statistics can only go so far. It is also critical to have a better understanding of how restrictive practices are experienced by people with disabilities and the interventions that can simultaneously maintain their safety, dignity and autonomy. Griffith et al. (2013) stressed that the findings of even small qualitative studies may be picked up and amplified through scoping reviews and systemic analyses, thereby adding weight to the burgeoning body of overall, usually quantitative, research. Qualitative research that draws specifically on how restrictive practices are experienced in different settings, such as schools or day programmes, and that gives greater voice to people with a range of diagnoses or who are disadvantaged in multiples will add necessary nuance to policy and practice conversations. For example, while it could be reasonably anticipated that environmental adjustments would help to reduce the use of restrictive practices in both specialist disability accommodation and mainstream school settings, the particular modifications required are likely to differ. Similarly, as another example, non-restrictive interventions to improve nutritional intake may be very different for a person whose food choices are primarily influenced by limited mobility or sensory aversions compared to someone living with Prader Willi Syndrome (PWS).[1] Alongside robust descriptive

1 PWS is a genetic disorder that includes persistent and insatiable appetite, hyperphagia and hunger-related eating behaviours and characteristics (Muscogiuri et al., 2021).

statistics, qualitative research can provide the detailed insights needed to effectively design and target policy and practice interventions that endeavour to offer a more powerful case to inform practice through descriptions of lived experience and participants' lives.

Qualitative research offers more than nuance. It also holds transformative potential for people whose autonomy has been undermined by restrictive practices and the discourse that attempts to legitimate them. As McDonald et al. (2016) explained and as noted earlier, people with intellectual disabilities value the opportunity to participate in research because they value being able to help others; they want the results of the research to be shared broadly to allow their community to learn more about people with intellectual disabilities, and ultimately, utilise the information learned to improve the lives of people with intellectual disabilities. Also (as described above), the experience of restrictive practices can be profoundly damaging to an individual's sense of self and esteem. The opportunity for people with disabilities to tell their stories and promote alternative approaches through meaningful participation in research may offer an important counterpoint to such aversive experiences. Indeed, as people who have used mental health services, Roper et al. (2021, p.17) described their participation in restrictive practice research as '"speaking back" to clinical power, law and the academy'. At a structural level, more participatory research is necessary to shift the current discourse away from dominant occupational health and safety considerations that have justified and sustained the use of restrictive practices (Cortis et al., 2023) towards a more person-centred and genuinely therapeutic approaches.

We propose that the following areas of exploration be prioritised by researchers and pursued through inclusive qualitative designs:

- Phenomenological studies into how different people with disabilities experience restrictive practices and their alternatives across settings. It is critical to consider how restrictive practices and less restrictive alternatives affect peoples' well-being, development, social, economic and community participation.
- Grounded theory studies that delineate preventative and proactive alternatives to restrictive practices as well as how best to engage people with disabilities who have experienced restrictive practices in research and other decision-making forums.
- Inclusive experimental research is needed to determine which approaches can meaningfully reduce and eventually eliminate restrictive practices.

There are several limitations to existing research on the topic of reducing or eliminating restrictive practices. First, it tends to focus on organisational and professional interventions rather than those driven or codesigned by people with disabilities (McSherry & Maker, 2021). Second (as detailed earlier in this chapter), evaluative research has focused on services for people with mental illnesses or psychosocial disability, therefore failing to capture the range of contexts in which people with disabilities currently experience restrictive interventions. Third, the evidence base is not yet robust enough to chart a clear policy or practice approach to reduce, let alone eliminate, restrictive practices (Cortis et al., 2023; Gooding et al., 2020). Finally, when success in reducing restrictive practices is demonstrated, the actual felt benefits for people subject to those practices remain unclear. For example, some interventions aimed at reducing physical restraints have resulted in a concomitant increase in the use of chemical restraint (Gaskin et al., 2013).

Further experimental and quasi-experimental research is needed to help shift efforts and investment towards non-restrictive interventions that make real differences to people with disabilities. There are important indicators that service-level involvement of peers is both desired by service users and beneficial in reducing the use of restrictive practices. For example, studies from the United States (Croft & İsvan, 2015; Greenfield et al., 2008) showed that peer-led mental health respite services were associated with improved service user satisfaction and therapeutic outcomes compared to psychiatric inpatient admissions while reducing the need for environmental restrictions. Another example, from Australia, described the CHOICE project, which found that youth mental health service users who received a codesigned intervention with the support of a youth peer worker with lived experience, reported feeling more involved in treatment decisions compared to the comparison group, which led to increased satisfaction in the service (Simmons et al., 2017, 2018). We therefore suggest that emphasis be given to experimental research that considers the effectiveness of models involving people with disabilities in the reduction of restrictive practices, including individualised behaviour support, supported decision-making and peer support models.

It is important to note that people who are more vulnerable to restrictive practices may also be less likely to be included in codesigned research and policymaking. Restrictive practices exist in the context of entrenched power dynamics and discrimination faced by people with disabilities (Spivakovsky et al., 2023), which makes willing and meaningful participation in research and policymaking particularly challenging. Being labelled as someone who uses challenging behaviours can be stigmatising and acts as an additional barrier. It is essential that researchers and other professionals seeking to involve people with disabilities who have been subject to restrictive practices in decision-making forums use person-centred approaches to prevent and respond to any challenging behaviours that might arise during the course of their activities.

Conclusion

Our case study (at the start of this chapter) provided a brief overview of Henry who, over the years, had many comprehensive behaviour support plans, including clear planning to fade out the many restrictive practices he was subject to. Initially, the restrictive practices were implemented and increased for Henry over time to mitigate occupational health and safety (OHS) risks and perceived risks to the community. With the introduction of a new disability service, the harm being inflicted upon Henry by the seclusion and chemical restraints were recognised. Empathising with the magnitude of his experience and the personal impact of long-term isolation, lack of connection, poor quality of life and denial of human rights was the initial consideration in planning for his new service and supports. It was when the gravity of harms were recognised as damaging and dangerous to Henry and given equal consideration within the risk assessment that decisive steps were taken to reduce the restrictions placed upon him. With supports strongly focused on valuing Henry's rights and experience, he now has access to his kitchen, food and drink, goes out into the community with supports regularly, does activities at home and has experienced and enjoyed regular activities outside the walls of his accommodation. His team is energised by the positive changes for Henry and is focused on continuing to build his quality of life and reduce restrictions further.

This chapter has outlined the critical need for people with disabilities to be more meaningfully involved in research and policy-making related to restrictive practices. From our perspective of working with children, young people and adults who continue to experience restrictions across many aspects of their lives, we have highlighted the transformative potential of lived experience perspectives; perspectives that can shift the discourse surrounding restrictive practices and advance promising alternatives. This chapter has identified several priority areas for lived experience research and practical considerations to more meaningfully involve people with disabilities in the drive to reduce and eliminate restrictive practices.

Please note that the case studies described in this chapter are based on real experiences. Names and identifying details have been changed to protect individual privacy.

References

Aguilar, C., & Pūras, D. (2015, April 1). Discrimination against autistic persons, the rule rather than the exception – UN rights experts. United Nations Office of The High Commissioner for

Human Rights. https://www.ohchr.org/en/press-releases/2015/04/discrimination-against-autistic-persons-rule-rather-exception-un-rights

Anderberg, E., & South, M. (2021). Predicting Parent Reactions at Diagnostic Disclosure Sessions for Autism. J AUTISM DEV DISORD. https://doi.org/10.1007/s10803-020-04817-5

Ashworth, M., Palikara, O., & Van Herwegen, J. (2019). Comparing parental stress of children with neurodevelopmental disorders: The case of Williams syndrome, Down syndrome and autism spectrum disorders. *Journal of Applied Research in Intellectual Disabilities*, *32*(5), 1047–1057.

Bailey, S., Boddy, K., Briscoe, S., & Morris, C. (2015). Involving disabled children and young people as partners in research: A systematic review. *Child: Care, Health and Development*, *41*, 505–514. https://doi.org/10.1111/cch.12197

Baker, J., Kendal, S., Berzins, K., Canvin, K., Branthonne-Foster, S., McDougall, T., Goldson, B., Kellar, I., Wright, J., & Duxbury, J. (2022). Mapping review of interventions to reduce the use of restrictive practices in children and young people's institutional settings: The CONTRAST study. *Children & Society, 36,* 1351–1401. https://doi.org/10.1111/chso.12581

Bartlett, N., & Ellis, T. F. (2020). Interrogating sanctioned violence: A survey of parents/guardians of children with disabilities about restraint and seclusion in Manitoba's schools. *Canadian Journal of Disability Studies*, *9*(5), 122–155. https://doi.org/10.15353/cjds.v9i5.693

BBC. (2022, March 26). *Maidstone school placed autistic boys in restraint chairs.* https://www.bbc.com/news/uk-england-kent-60877569

Bisschops, E. H., de Schipper, J. C., Schippers, B., Embregts, P. J. C. M., & Schuengel, C. (2022). Reducing restrictive measures in complex long-term care for people with intellectual disabilities: Implementation interventions through the lens of normalisation process theory. *Journal of Intellectual & Developmental Disability*, 1–12. https://doi.org/10.3109/13668250.2022.2044270

Björne, P., Deveau, R., McGill, P., & Nylander, L. (2022), The use of restrictive measures in community services for people with intellectual disabilities in Sweden. *Journal of Policy and Practice in Intellectual Disabilities, 19*(2), 193–201. https://doi.org/10.1111/jppi.12399

Brophy, L. M., Roper, C. E., Hamilton, B. E., Tellez, J. J., & McSherry, B. M. (2016). Consumers' and their supporters' perspectives on barriers and strategies to reducing seclusion and restraint in mental health settings. *Australian Health Review: A publication of the Australian Hospital Association, 40*(6), 599–604. https://doi.org/10.1071/AH15128

Carter, W. (2006) Challenging Behaviour and Disability: A Targeted Response. *Report to Honourable Warren Pitt M.P. Minister for Communities Disability Services and Seniors.*

Children and Young People with Disability Australia. (2016, July 16). *Submission to the Special Rapporteur on the rights of persons with disability: Abuse of students with disability in Australian schools.* https://cyda.org.au/abuse-of-students-with-disability-in-australian-schools/

CNN. (2011, January 23). *Case of young man tied to wall sparks national debate in Netherlands.* http://edition.cnn.com/2011/WORLD/europe/01/22/netherlands.documentary/index.html

Commonwealth of Australia (2023, September 29). Royal Commission into violence, abuse, neglect and exploitation of people with disability: Final report: Volume 6: Enabling autonomy and access. (Updated November 2). https://disability.royalcomission.gov.au/publications/final-report

Connolly, A. (Reporter). (2023, September 25). Careless (Season 2023, Episode 28) [Tv series episode]. In M. Carney (Executive Producer), *Four corners.* Australian Broadcasting Corporation.

Cortis, N., Smyth, C. & Katz, I. (2023). Reducing restrictive practices: A review of evidence-based alternatives. Report for the Royal Commission into Violence, Abuse, Neglect and Exploitation of People with Disability. UNSW Social Policy Research Centre.

Croft, B., & İsvan, N. (2015). Impact of the 2nd story peer respite program on use of inpatient and emergency services. *Psychiatric Services, 66*(6), 632–637. https://doi.org/10.1176/appi.ps.201400266

Damiano, C. R., Mazefsky, C. A., White, S. W., & Dichter, G. S. (2014). Future Directions for Research in Autism Spectrum Disorders. J Clin Child Adolesc Psychol, 43(5), 828–843. https://doi.org/10.1080/15374416.2014.945214

Dean, E. E., Fisher, K. W., Shogren, K. A., & Wehmeyer, M. L. (2016). Participation and Intellectual Disability: A Review of the Literature. Intellectual and Developmental Disabilities, 54(6), 427–439. https://doi.org/10.1352/1934-9556-54.6.427

Department of Health. (2023, June 23*). Developing a strategy towards elimination of seclusion and restraint.* https://www.health.vic.gov.au/mental-health-wellbeing-reform/developing-a-strategy-towards-elimination-of-seclusion-and-restraint

Downes, N., Lichtlé, J., Lamore, K., Orêve, M. J., & Cappe, E. (2020). Couples' Experiences of Parenting a Child After an Autism Diagnosis: A Qualitative Study. Journal of autism and developmental disorders. https://doi.org/10.1007/s10803-020-04744-5

Ferguson, P. M., & Nusbaum, E. (2012). Disability studies: What is it and what difference does it make? *Research and Practice for Persons with Severe Disabilities*, *37*(2), 70–80. https://doi.org/10.1177/154079691203700202

Fitton, L., & Jones, D. R. (2020). Restraint of adults with intellectual disabilities: A critical review of the prevalence and characteristics associated with its use. *Journal of Intellectual Disabilities*, *24*(2), 268–283. https://doi.org/10.1177/1744629518778695

Flinders University and Council for Intellectual Disability. (n.d.). *Deciding with support*. https://decidingwithsupport.flinders.edu.au

Franks, Z. M., Alcock, J. A., Lam, T., Haines, K. J., Arora, N., & Ramanan, M. (2021). Physical restraints and post-traumatic stress disorder in survivors of critical illness. A systematic review and meta-analysis. *Annals of the American Thoracic Society*, *18*(4), 689–697.

Gaskin, C. J., McVilly, K. R., & McGillivray, J. A. (2013). Initiatives to reduce the use of seclusion and restraints on people with developmental disabilities: A systematic review and quantitative synthesis. *Research in Developmental Disabilities*, *34*(11), 3946–3961. https://doi.org/10.1016/j.ridd.2013.08.010

Giri, A., Aylott, J., Giri, P., Ferguson-Wormley, S., & Evans, J. (2022). Lived experience and the social model of disability: Conflicted and inter-dependent ambitions for employment of people with a learning disability and their family carers. *British Journal of Learning Disabilities*, *50*(1), 98–106.

Gooding, P., McSherry, B., & Roper, C. (2020). Preventing and reducing 'coercion' in mental health services: an international scoping review of English-language studies. *Acta Psychiatrica Scandinavia*, *142*, 27–39. https://doi.org/10.1111/acps.13152

Greenfield, T.K., Stoneking, B.C., Humphreys, K., Sundby, E. and Bond, J. (2008). A randomized trial of a mental health consumer-managed alternative to civil commitment for acute psychiatric crisis. *American Journal of Community Psychology*, *42*, 135–144. https://doi.org/10.1007/s10464-008-9180-1

Griffith, G. M., Hutchinson, L., & Hastings, R. P. (2013). "I'm not a patient, I'm a person": The experiences of individuals with intellectual disabilities and challenging behaviour - A thematic synthesis of qualitative studies. *Clinical Psychology: Science and Practice*, *20*(4), 469. https://doi.org/10.1111/cpsp.12053

Hayward, B. A., McKay-Brown, L., & Poed, S. (2022). Restrictive practices and the 'need' for positive behaviour support (PBS): A critical discourse examination of disability policy beliefs. *Journal of Intellectual Disabilities*, *27*(1), 170–189. https://doi.org/10.1177/17446295211062383

Huang, Y., Arnold, S. R. C., Foley, K.-R., & Trollor, J. N. (2020). Diagnosis of autism in adulthood: A scoping review. Autism, 24(6), 1311–1327. https://doi.org/10.1177/1362361320903128

Hughes, O. (2023). Pedagogies of lived experience: The perspectives of people with disabilities on their educational presentations about disability topics. Disability Studies Quarterly, 42(3–4). https://doi.org/10.18061/dsq.v42i3-4.8120

Hui, A., Middleton, H., & Völlm, B. (2016). The uses of coercive measures in forensic psychiatry: A literature review. In B. Völlm & N. Nedopil (Eds.), *The use of coercive measures in forensic psychiatric care: Legal, ethical and practical challenges*, 151–184. Springer.

Jacobs, D., Steyaert, J., Dierickx, K., & Hens, K. (2020). Parents' views and experiences of the autism spectrum disorder diagnosis of their young child: a longitudinal interview study. European child & adolescent psychiatry, 29(8), 1143–1154. https://doi.org/10.1007/s00787-019-01431-4

Jones, S. C., Akram, M., Gordon, C. S., Murphy, N., & Sharkie, F. (2021). Autism in Australia: Community Knowledge and Autistic People's Experiences. Journal of autism and developmental disorders, 51(10), 3677–3689. https://doi.org/10.1007/s10803-020-04819-3

Kinner, S. A., Harvey, C., Hamilton, B., Brophy, L., Roper, C., McSherry, B., & Young, J. T. (2017). Attitudes towards seclusion and restraint in mental health settings: findings from a large, community-based survey of consumers, carers and mental health professionals. *Epidemiology and Psychiatric Sciences*, *26*(5), 535–544. https://doi.org/10.1017/S2045796016000585

Leif, E., Fox, R., Subban, P., & Sharma, U. (2023). 'Stakeholders are almost always resistant': Australian behaviour support practitioners' perceptions of the barriers and enablers to reducing restrictive practices. *International Journal of Developmental Disabilities*, *69*(1), 66–82. https://doi.org/10.1080/20473869.2022.2116908

Lennox, N., Taylor, M., Rey-Conde, T., Bain, C., Purdie, D. M., & Boyle, F. (2005). Beating the barriers: recruitment of people with intellectual disability to participate in research. Journal of Intellectual Disability Research, 49(4), 296–305. https://doi.org/10.1111/j.1365-2788.2005.00618.x

Matson, J. L., & Shoemaker, M. (2009). Intellectual disability and its relationship to autism spectrum disorders. Research in developmental disabilities, 30(6), 1107–1114. https://doi.org/10.1016/j.ridd.2009.06.003

McDonald, K. E., Conroy, N. E., & Olick, R. S. (2016). Is It Worth It? Benefits in Research With Adults With Intellectual Disability. Intellectual and Developmental Disabilities, 54(6), 440–453. https://doi.org/10.1352/1934-9556-54.6.440

McLean, S., & Halstead, E. J. (2021). Resilience and stigma in mothers of children with emotional and behavioural difficulties. *Research in Developmental Disabilities, 108*, 103818. https://doi.org/10.1016/j.ridd.2020.103818

McSherry, B., & Maker, Y. (2021). Restrictive practices: Options and opportunities. In B. McSherry & Y. Maker (Eds.), *Restrictive practices in health care and disability settings: Legal, policy and practical responses* (pp. 2–15). Routledge.

Meehan, T., Vermeer, C., & Windsor, C. (2000). Patients' perceptions of seclusion: A qualitative investigation. *Journal of Advanced Nursing, 31*(2), 370–377.

Ministers for the Department of Social Services. (2024, July 31). *Government response to the Disability Royal Commission.* Dss.gov.au. https://ministers.dss.gov.au/media-releases/15471

Muscogiuri, G., Barrea, L., Faggiano, F., Maiorino, M. I., Parrillo, M., Pugliese, G., Ruggeri, R. M., Scarano, E., Savastano, S., & Colao, A. (2021). Obesity in Prader–Willi syndrome: physiopathological mechanisms, nutritional and pharmacological approaches. *Journal of Endocrinological Investigation, 44*(10), 2057–2070. https://doi.org/10.1007/s40618-021-01574-9

Nunno, M.A., McCabe, L.A., Izzo, C.V., Smith, E.G., Sellers, D.E., & Holden, M.J. (2022). A 26-year study of restraint fatalities among children and adolescents in the United States: A failure of organizational structures and processes. *Child & Youth Care Forum, 51*, 661–680. https://doi.org/10.1007/s10566-021-09646-w

Perkins, R., Rinaldi, M., & Hardisty, J. (2010). Harnessing the expertise of experience: Increasing access to employment within mental health services for people who have themselves experienced mental health problems. *Diversity in Health and Care 7*, 13–21.

Poed, S., Cologon, K., & Jackson, R. (2020). Gatekeeping and restrictive practices by Australian mainstream schools: Results of a national survey. *International Journal of Inclusive Education, 26*(8), 766–779. https://doi.org/10.1080/13603116.2020.1726512

Poslawsky, I. E., Poslawsky, I. E., Naber, F. B. A., Naber, F. B. A., Van Daalen, E., Van Daalen, E., Van Engeland, H., & Van Engeland, H. (2014). Parental Reaction to Early Diagnosis of Their Children's Autism Spectrum Disorder: An Exploratory Study. Child Psychiatry Hum Dev, 45(3), 294–305. https://doi.org/10.1007/s10578-013-0400-z

Ramcharan, P., Nankervis, K., Strong, T., & Robertson, A. (2009). *Experiences of restrictive practices: A view from people with disabilities and family carers.*

Rasmussen, P. S., Pedersen, I. K., & Pagsberg, A. K. (2020). Biographical disruption or cohesion? How parents deal with their child's autism diagnosis. Soc Sci Med, 244, 112673–112673. https://doi.org/10.1016/j.socscimed.2019.112673

Reed, P., & Osborne, L. A. (2019). Reaction to diagnosis and subsequent health in mothers of children with autism spectrum disorder. Autism, 23(6), 1442–1448. https://doi.org/10.1177/1362361318815641

Richardson, B., Webber, L. S., & Lambrick, F. (2019). Factors associated with long-term use of restrictive interventions. *Journal of*

Intellectual & Developmental Disability, *45*(2), 159–166. https://doi.org/10.3109/13668250.2019.1639895

Ridley, J., & Leitch, S. (2021). Restraint Reduction Network training standards: First edition. British Institute of Learning Disabilities. https://restraintreductionnetwork.org/wp-content/uploads/2023/10/RRN_standards_v9_accessible_PDF_updated.pdf

Roper, C., O'Hagan, M., Kennedy, H., & Roennfeldt, H. (2021). Ending restraint: An insider view. In B. McSherry & Y. Maker (Eds.), *Restrictive practices in health care and disability settings: Legal, policy and practical responses* (pp. 16–38). Routledge.

Røstad, M., Whittington, R., & Søndenaa, E. (2023). Minimising restrictive interventions for people with an intellectual disability: Documentary analysis of decisions to reduce coercion in Norway. *Scandinavian Journal of Disability Research*, *25*(1), 160–169. https://doi.org/10.16993/sjdr.984

Schippers, B., Frederiks, B. J., van Nieuwenhuijzen, M., & Schuengel, C. (2018). Reliability and feasibility of systematic registration of coercive measures in care for people with intellectual disabilities. *Journal of Policy and Practice in Intellectual Disabilities, 15*(3), 202–213.

Simmons, M. B., Batchelor, S., Dimopoulos-Bick, T., & Howe, D. (2017). The choice project: peer workers promoting shared decision making at a youth mental health service. *Psychiatric services, 68*(8), 764–770.

Simmons, M. B., Coates, D., Batchelor, S., Dimopoulos-Bick, T., & Howe, D. (2018). The CHOICE pilot project: Challenges of implementing a combined peer work and shared decision-making programme in an early intervention service. *Early intervention in psychiatry*, *12*(5), 964–971.

Spivakovsky, C., Steele, L., & Wadiwel, D. (2023). *Restrictive practices: A pathway to elimination.* Commonwealth of Australia Royal Commission into violence, abuse, neglect and exploitation of people with a disability. https://disability.royalcommission.gov.au/system/files/2023-07/Research%20Report%20-%20Restrictive%20practices%20-%20A%20pathway%20to%20elimination.pdf

State of Victoria, 2021. Royal Commission into Victoria's Mental Health System: Final Report (PP No 202, Session 2018–2021 (document 1 of 6), Issue.

United Nations. (2006). *Convention on the rights of people with disabilities – Articles.* https://social.desa.un.org/issues/disability/crpd/convention-on-the-rights-of-persons-with-disabilities-articles

United Nations. (2023). *Progress on disability rights risks going in reverse: Guterres*. Retrieved May 7, 2024, from https://social.desa.un.org/issues/disability/news/progress-on-disability-rights-risks-going-in-reverse-guterres

Willis, J., Harrison, A., & Allen, J.L. (2021). Pupils with social, emotional and mental health special needs: Perceptions of how restrictive physical interventions impact their relationships with teaching staff. *Teaching and Teacher Education*, *97*, 103219. https://doi.org/10.1016/j.tate.2020.103219

World Health Organisation and The World Bank. (2017). *Model disability survey: Survey manual.* https://iris.who.int/bitstream/handle/10665/258513/9789241512862-eng.pdf?sequence=1

Younan, B., Jorgensen, M., Chan, J., Winata, T., & Gillies, D. (2024). Restrictive practice use in people with neurodevelopmental disorders: A systematic review. *Advances in Neurodevelopmental Disorders, 8*(1), 122–140.

4
Policies to address information deprivation for people with disability

Cassandra Wright-Dole

Introduction

In 2023, the Australian Government published the final report of the *Royal Commission into Violence, Abuse, Neglect and Exploitation of People with Disability* (Disability Royal Commission [DRC]). A key finding from the DRC was that '[accessible] information and communications are a critical safeguard against violence, abuse, neglect, and exploitation' and 'are necessary for people with disability to exercise autonomy' (Commonwealth of Australia, 2023, p.39). This finding underlines the crucial role accessible information (AI) can play in safeguarding people and their well-being. The term *accessible information* is defined as '... information which is able to be read or received and understood by the individual or group for which it is intended' (NHS England, 2015) and encompasses many different inclusive formats such as braille, large print, audio description, live captioning and so forth. AI is generally an umbrella term for all forms of information that positions accessibility at the forefront of its delivery; however, for this chapter, it refers to written content that is designed to be readable, comprehensible and actionable for individuals with low literacy to counteract information deprivation resulting from low literacy challenges.

In emphasising the significant role that AI can play in protecting against harm, the DRC has also drawn attention to the reality that 'many people with disability in Australia still cannot access information and communications on an equal basis with others' (Commonwealth of Australia, 2023, p. 50). Historically, public institutions have been spaces that have been situated as 'safe' spaces or spaces that are 'informed' about how to work with people with disabilities. On the contrary, people with disability, according to the Council for Intellectual Disability (2023), 'often find information and communications inaccessible, in contexts including health care, disability service settings like group homes, education, employment, and prisons' (*Accessible information and communications*, 2023).

Accessible information is often understood as an accommodation that is legally required for people with disability under human rights law (Meltzer, 2020, p. 478) or viewed as a necessity for a minority that 'does not attain a functional level of literacy skills' (Basterfield, 2019, p. 19). However, low literacy is the recurrent theme of the need for accessible information making accessible information formats, such as Easy English, increasingly relevant to a wide audience (Basterfield, 2019, p. 17).

In this chapter, I argue that persistent exposure to inaccessible information, not low literacy, precedes information deprivation and disrupts the social participation of those with low literacy. This chapter examines the prevalence of low literacy and how linguicism excludes people with low literacy from effective autonomous social participation, comparing it to the lived experience of a profoundly deaf person who does not have a natural sign language. After describing my lived experience of linguistic and information discrimination, I introduce the theory of atypical linguicism as a form of linguicism concerned with the relationship between expectations of ability and resultant linguistic exclusion and information deprivation. Following a brief overview and critical analysis of written AI formats available in Australia, this chapter concludes with policy and research recommendations for a path forward.

The global prevalence of literacy: Accessible information implications for social participation and inclusion

The Organisation for Economic Co-operation and Development (OECD) defines literacy as 'the ability to understand and utilise printed information in daily activities, at home, at work, and in the community—to achieve one's goals and to develop one's knowledge and potential' (2000, p. x). This definition of literacy extends beyond reading proficiency to encompass functional understanding and application, recognising that individuals with low literacy will likely encounter difficulties in everyday reading tasks. Literacy is typically measured according to the International Standard Classification of Education 2011 (ISCED, 2012), which can be condensed into three corresponding levels:

- ISCED 0–2: *Low education;*
- ISCED 3–4: *Medium education; and*
- ISCED 5–8: *High education*

Globally, more than 750 million people 15 years of age or older are deemed to have literacy skills at or below ISCED level 2 (UNESCO, 2017), indicating a need for AI across a significant proportion of the global population. This statistic indicates a significant global policy challenge within developed and developing nations. Moving forward, AI is needed to mitigate the effects of low literacy on social participation and inclusion. For example, Garcia et al. highlight the association between low literacy and a poor understanding of medical information, an association that ultimately has 'implications for the quality and costs of healthcare for patients with low health literacy' (2010, p. 65). Beyond difficulty with reading, comprehension or utilising written information appropriately, low literacy tacitly weakens the individual's core knowledge base due to reduced access to information from the outset.

In present-day Australia, literacy is critical for individual participation in private, social and public life. However, while literacy is necessary for people's ability to access information, accessible information cannot be discounted as a viable means to mitigate systematic exclusion and subsequent poor outcomes associated with low literacy. Failure to provide a person with low literacy access to information in a way they can understand is tantamount to refusing a non-native speaker access to translated information. Such exclusion is a form of language discrimination known as linguicism.

Linguicism and social exclusion

Linguicism was first defined by sociolinguist Tove Skutnabb-Kangas as 'ideologies, structures and practices which are used to legitimate, effectuate, regulate and reproduce an unequal division of power and resources' (1986, p. 41). This ideology is shared by other theorists such as Pierre Bourdieu, a French sociologist, who viewed language as a signifier of social stratification and a mechanism of power (1991), and Michel Foucault, a French historian and philosopher, who saw language as a tool of the powerful to construct knowledge and truths as a means of social control (1998). This concept of language as power can be derived from its centrality to society, as both contemporary and historical social phenomena, and its systematic weaponisation throughout the time when language was used to keep the 'othered' subordinate (Fairclough, 1989; Bryan & Herrera, 2023).

Such underpinnings of linguicism are not limited to language bias or dialectical snobbery but also extend to exclusion from linguistic participation through inaccessible modes of communication. Crip Theory engages with intersectionality from the shared perspective and experience of the role normativity plays within power relations. At the centre of this intersectionality is the invisibility of the 'normal' (Karlsson & Rydstrom, 2023). In Crip Theory, it is able-bodiedness (McRuer, 2006); in queer theory, it is heteronormativity (Kafer, 2013); and in critical race theory, it is whiteness (Morris, 2016). This shared concept between minority-centred ideologies focuses on the contrast in attitudes when distinctions are drawn between the 'othered' and the 'normal', with normativity seen as the ideal to marginalise those that deviate from the norm. Certain inherent characteristics and aspects relating to social status (such as socioeconomic status) exist as normate; *normate* is defined as 'an idealised position that has dominance and authority in society' (Garland-Thomson, 1997, p. 8). Able-bodiedness is one form of normate; literate is another. The concept of able-bodiedness within Crip Theory is not only thought to define disability, but it is also deemed responsible for creating disability through default provision for ability overall. In this context, society sets the stage for information deprivation when it fails to make information accessible to those who experience low literacy. This is evident when I consider the lived experience of linguistic and information deprivation, as has been the case in my lived experience of deafness.

My lived experience of linguistic and information deprivation

In the late 1980s, I lost most of my hearing in over a period of six months. By the time I was 7 years old, I was profoundly deaf:

> This child has suffered a progressive hearing loss and is now close to being totally deaf... and indeed will be lucky to remain in the normal school system if further deterioration occurs." (H. Rundle, personal communication, August 1988).

Determined not to let me fall through the cracks, my parents encouraged me to continue communicating, as I had before, with a suspected mild hearing loss, through lipreading and speaking. There is no manual for raising children, let alone one for raising a child with a disability, and my parents did the best they could with what information they had at the time. Guided by state education policies, my parents were eager to follow recommendations of best practices.

In the 1980s, the world had not progressed in understanding the psychology of deafness or disability to the extent it has today. To be a close fit to 'normal' was considered best practice under the accepted medical model of disability. The medical model of disability focuses on disability as a malfunction of the individual, designating it as the root cause of any problems arising from being disabled. It ignores societal barriers, instead focusing on the disability as the barrier to successful independent social participation (Australian Federation of Disability Organisations, 2025). For this reason, many parents of d/Deaf children received rigid instructions about how to approach language development: 'We were told that we should sit on our hands and not use any kind of sign or gesture. The sole means of communication would be through lipreading…' (a research participant in Payne et al., 2022, p. 76).

Skuttnabb-Kangas refers to this mentality as *audism*, a form of linguicism directed at deafness (Skuttnabb-Kangas, 1986; Phillipson, 2012). Audism fosters the idea of deafness as an anomaly to be minimised in favour of conformity in the hearing world. It sets the expectations for d/Deaf people to achieve hearing-centred norms (Humphrey & Alcorn, 1995). It also fosters the belief that listening is superior to other linguistic modes and modalities of receiving information, such as sign language. This belief continues to be prevalent within many societies; speech is the 'normal' linguistic modality and should be adhered to at all costs. For far too long, this view has denied deaf children access to language and education, negating their ability to access information and exposing them to information deprivation.

Such attitudes were reflected in the insistence that I practice using my residual hearing.

> [Her] listening skills have shown improvement, but [she] has a negative attitude still to listening skills activities with [the visiting teacher], but this is still a priority (Integration Support Group, personal communication, 16 May, 1989).

I remember a fluorescent light and a small brown-haired boy. His hands moved deftly, his smile earnest, his voice inaudible – if not by my deafness, his own. As a mirror image of my sensory constraints sat across from me in the waiting room, I can remember the intense joy I felt to not be alone in my silence. I understood his hand movements as much as I could understand speech, but it did not matter:

> Cassie [is] rather unsettled at the moment; wonders when her ears will get better.... Questioning why she, and not others, has become deaf (Integration Support Group, personal communication, 15 March, 1988).
> Teacher report to Integration Support Group, 15 March 1988

All that had mattered when I was playing with the small brown-haired boy was the fleeting sensation of ordinariness that I had experienced.

Once back home, I stubbornly refused to speak, instead moving my hands around nonsensically as I tried to position myself in a place of belonging. My parents' reaction to my self-imposed silence was both swift and effective. Although they never intended to insinuate that my differences were best unseen, the eagerness of adults to praise me for not embodying my deafness juxtaposed against the clear message that I was not to identify as a non-speaking 'capital D' Deaf person was quickly absorbed by my young mind. My mother did take me to sign language classes not long after; however, rather than embrace the opportunity, I stoically told her I was 'not one of those Deaf people', and that was the end of that.

Oralism, like audism, is a form of linguicism that others deafness. It results in d/Deaf people being expected to speak and labelled deficient compared to their hearing and speaking counterparts when they cannot (Kusters & Lucas, 2022, p. 89). This form of linguicism rejects sign language outright in favour of listening and speech, often requiring the d/Deaf person to undergo extensive therapies contrary to their abilities (Mathews, 2017, p. 3). According to Kusters and Lucas, oralism existed as early as the nineteenth century and has long resulted in professionals routinely discouraging parents from promoting sign language use in their children (2022, p. 89).

I was in grade one when my mother and my integration aide pushed for sign language again, asking for a sign language teacher to come to the school so that I would be learning with my hearing peers and there would be another means of communication accessible to me. The visiting teacher said I would benefit from my peers learning sign language alongside me.

The benefits would be better quality communication between myself and others in the school community; it would alleviate the high degree of concentration required by lipreading and promote social participation and well-being. Then, underlined in bright red ink:

> Signing must, at all times, be accompanied by speech. Cass must not sign without speaking. She is not obligated to sign herself"(Integration Support Group, personal communication, 14 September, 1988).

After discovering this school correspondence, I messaged my childhood integration aide. Soon after exchanging pleasantries, I began questioning her about why signing during Auslan had not been mandatory for me. She seemed confused at first but explained that instead of Auslan, I was taught Signed English. Some years ago, I learned that Auslan has a different grammatical structure from English, and I often wondered why my signing lexicon included certain words, such as 'is', 'to' and 'the'.

In the weeks following the introduction of sign language in my classroom, the teacher had reported, 'Sign language has been a big help for Cassie with her peers' (Teacher report to Integration Support Group, personal communication, 26 October, 1988).

The realisation that while I thought I was learning to sign like 'my people', I had not been learning their language at all hit hard. Could it explain why many of my interactions with Deaf children had seemed just as complicated as with hearing children? Just as my 'spoken' voice was othered in the hearing world, my 'sign' voice had been 'lacking' in the Deaf world. Despite the benefits of the communicative repertoire reported by my teacher, the inclusion of Signed English in the classroom was abandoned within 2 years of starting:

> It has been found that signing as a form of communication is not necessary, and instruction in this area has ceased (Integration Support Group, personal communication, 15 August, 1990).

The correspondence from the meeting did not specify reasons, but Signed English functions as a sign system to bolster English language skills by reinforcing grammar and syntax (National Deaf Children's Society, 2025; Scott & Henner, 2021), and according to the school report of the same year, my literacy met the expected level. The new focus for my integration was to improve my residual hearing and ensure 'equal access to information' for me as a 'hearing-impaired' student (Integration Support Group, personal communication, 15 August, 1990).

The role of atypical linguicism in information deprivation

In my ongoing research, I propose a new theory I call atypical linguicism. *Atypical linguicism* is a phenomenon that relates to an individual's ability to engage with linguistic modes (speaking, writing, listening and reading) rather than meeting expectations of linguistic competence. It may be defined as language discrimination, that is, consciously or unconsciously, directed towards people unable to utilise specific forms or modes of communication for reasons beyond their control, such as physical, sensory or intellectual disabilities, learning disorders or socio-economic barriers. Atypical linguicism is present in interactions or engagements with people who face barriers in communication due to an atypical semiotic repertoire rather than the language in which it is communicated. The *semiotic repertoire* is 'the totality of semiotic resources that people use when they communicate (such as speech, image, text, gesture, sign, gaze, facial expression, posture, objects and so on)' (Kusters, 2021, p. 183). As such, atypical linguicism relates to the expectation of linguistic assimilation regarding the ability to utilise semiotic sources rather than the language itself. For example, the American Library Association based in the United States defines *information literacy* as having the capacity to 'recognise when information is needed and have the ability to locate, evaluate, and use effectively the needed information' (1989). For people experiencing low literacy, the inability to effectively engage with information written for the public inherently forms the basis of the individual's exclusion from social participation. For example, to engage with and obtain support from government agencies, such as health, legal or financial services, people are typically provided with written information and required to complete forms. For those with low literacy, this can present an insurmountable barrier. Inaccessible information may preclude people from:

a. Accessing government support.
b. Understanding their rights and obligations (e.g. local bylaws).
c. Understanding contracts and providing informed consent (e.g. rental agreements).
d. Understanding medical conditions or how to take medication (OECD, 2000).

The foundation of atypical linguicism is heavily derived from Jonathon Henner and Octavian Robinson's Crip Linguistics theory that language is dependent on bodies. The term 'crip' has had long-held derogatory connotations, but has since been reclaimed by disability groups and consequently adopted into critical disability theory's lexicon. The renewed use of the word seeks to redefine the current status quo and forge a transformative path forward (Henner & Robinson, 2023a). However, not all share the optimism about this extension of disability theory. Bone (2017) argues that crip theory silences the disabled experience and fails to address the gaping chasm between theory and the lived reality of disability, while Jenks (2019) believes that the assumption of a unified disabled identity poses problematic in understanding the politics of disability and the failure of 'crip identity' to acknowledge the role of impairment in disability politics. This focus shares similarities with Bone (2017) concerning the implications of denying people with disabilities a voice but from the failure to differentiate between the disabled experience of impairment.

'Crip theory' conceptualises the intersectionality of disability and queerness through recognition of their thematic similarities in identity politics. Exploring queer and disabled identities in 'Feminist Queer Crip', Kafer views crip theory through the lens of the typical mainstream view of heterosexuality and able-bodiedness as the status quo (2013). They argue that the queer and disabled identities exist as a construct of difference. These views echo the sentiment of McRuer: 'Able-bodiedness, even more than heterosexuality, still largely masquerades as a non-identity, as the natural order of things' (2006, p. 1). Those who cannot secure a non-identity are identified by their inherent traits within society, which provide them with the identity of 'other', an identity of difference.

The underlying argument for atypical linguicism aligns with Critical Disability Theory, which puts forward that people with disability experience oppression within similar contexts to those who experience racism and other forms of cultural, historical, social and political oppression (Hall, 2019). Atypical linguicism embraces the notion of intersectionality within crip theory due to vulnerable minorities sharing the experience of being 'othered'. As with able-bodiedness, functional literacy is considered normate within Australia and other Western countries. This phenomenon supports the need to expand the context of the social conditions that contribute to the lack of accessible information made available to those with stigmatised attributes.

Margrit Shildrick, an Emeritus professor in Critical Disability Studies, explores the shift from rehabilitation perspectives toward pragmatic solutions, but highlights the need to deconstruct normative assumptions within the societal narrative of disability (2012). She further characterises the coexistence of 'the formal integration of disabled people into the standard rights, obligations, and expectations of normative citizenship' as a failure to deconstruct the perception of disability as exceptional (Shildrick, 2012, p. 2). Atypical linguicism shares Shildrick's observations on these conventions. It likens the deconstruction of normative assumptions necessary for removing the presumption of literacy when creating information for public dissemination. Additionally, it views the need to deconstruct the perception of disability as exceptional, instead manifesting the need for a universal design approach to information to normalise inclusion and accessibility in information.

Crip theory calls for a greater understanding of how people with disability experience aspects of life in contradiction with the experience of non-disabled people. For example, Kafer explores the concept of crip time, which explores how people with disabilities experience or relate to time (2013, p. 25). Kafer, like Shildrick, calls for the deconstruction of the normative through 'reimagining our notions of what can or should happen in time', viewing the focus on cure and referral as framing disability as a failure (Kafer, 2013, p. 27). In context with information, a focus on adult literacy programmes to address low literacy or presume that a support worker will support a person with a disability to know required information continues to 'bend' the person with the disability rather than addressing the issue of inaccessible information. Failure to address this issue gives rise to social inequities, such as poorer health or exclusion from accessing government supports.

The third principle, in Henner and Robinson's Crip Linguistics, states that 'Disability in languaging cannot be separated from normative expectations of language use' (Henner & Robinson, 2023, p. 1), suggesting that stigma exists with the deviance from normative linguistic expectations beyond the scope of raciolinguistics. *Raciolinguistics* focuses on the relationship between language and race. For example, where standardised English exists as a denominator for social inclusion, the standardisation serves to marginalise those whose linguistic practices fail to meet those standards; this extends to linguistic practices deemed not only foreign but also deviant, such as dialect, accent or inflections

(Alim et al., 2016, p. 165). One of the more apparent perceived deviances associated with a disability is multimodal approaches to languaging; for example, sign language deviates from the heavily misguided presumption that speech (and only speech) is normative. Therefore, those who use sign language may have their language marked as disordered. Other multimodal ways of languaging viewed as disordered may also be intrinsically interwoven with a disability that removes the presumption of speech, such as Augmented and Alternative Communication (AAC). Crip linguistics inherently resists the view that there is only one way to language (Henner & Robinson, 2023a, p.15).

Similarly, atypical linguicism argues that limited access to information rather than an individual's perceived linguistic deficiencies creates barriers to accessing essential public information, for example, health information or information about their rights. As such, the barrier to information is created by social expectations of ability, which are incorporated into information formats, including many AI formats. Much AI becomes unnecessarily inaccessible to a large proportion of the intended audience in the context of public information.

Critical discussion of three dominant types of accessible information in Australia

The issue of inaccessible public information is a product of the systematic entrenchment of linguicism within public institution processes. It is in direct conflict with human rights instruments that Australia is a signatory to. In the Convention on the Rights of

Persons with Disabilities (CRPD), two articles are specifically relevant to the issue of accessible information – Article 9 and Article 21. Article 9 relates the right of people with disabilities to 'live independently and participate fully in all aspects of life', highlighting the responsibility of the state to act to 'include the identification and elimination of obstacles and barriers to accessibility,' including in regard to Section 1 (b): information, communications and other services, including electronic services and emergency services (United Nations, 2006, Article 9). Article 21 mandates that information provided for the public should be available 'to persons with disabilities in accessible formats and technologies appropriate to different kinds of disabilities in a timely manner and without additional cost' (United Nations, 2006, Article 21), providing people with information in a way that they can understand is a human right that honours their autonomy and right to make informed choices.

Accessible information formats are language varieties with reduced linguistic complexity that 'aim to improve readability and comprehensibility' (Hansen-Schirra & Maaβ, 2020, p. 17). However, the appropriate language variety within written communication remains increasingly subjective, with each of the written formats having their supporters and critics, and then further division within those that support the use of the same formats.

In Australia, the three dominant types of accessible information are *Plain Language, Easy Read and Easy English.*

Plain Language

Plain Language is 'an approach to language and design for producing accessible and readable public documents' (Matveeva et al., 2017, p. 336). According to the Plain Language Association International, Plain Language requires careful consideration of the audience and the purpose of the information. It should use a logical structure familiar to the target audience, supportive visual elements in the design, careful use of syntax and evaluation of readability for the audience before dissemination (Plain Language Association International, 2025). Willerton argues that Plain Language is a response that affords people access to their rights, combatting 'the information apartheid that convoluted, overly complicated documents generate' (2015, p. xiii).

Easy Read

The Australian Government Style Manual classifies Easy Read as suitable for 4–6-year olds (Digital Transformation Agency, 2021; Australian Bureau of Statistics, 2013b). According to Buell et al., Easy Read refers to large print documents with simple language and are typically supported by a visual cue such as a photo, icon or image (2020, p. 220). Hurtado defines Easy Read as the construction of 'information in a way that is easy for the recipient to understand' and states that it 'exceeds simply simplifying the vocabulary and grammar' (2014, p. 823); it is this that differentiates Easy Read from Plain Language. Townsley et al. (2003) promote simplification processes such as short sentences, one idea per sentence and the use of active tense when creating accessible information. It also underscores the importance of direct and consistent language and using examples to help the reader process the information. These characteristics are important to allow the reader to understand the information and assist them in putting the information into practical use.

Easy English

Easy English material is broken down to show one idea and supports the concept using a concrete image (Basterfield, 2019). According to Scope, one of the largest not-for-profit disability services providers in Australia, Easy English aims to introduce key information to the reader through the removal of non-essential details (2015). Specific features are 'simplified language and grammar, minimal punctuation, simplified font, layout and design, and images that illustrate headings and key messages' (Scope, 2015, p. 2). The earlier definition of accessible text by Townsley et al. (2003) aligns with Plain Language and Easy Read rather than Easy English. In contrast, Basterfield outlines Easy English as having shorter sentences, using the consumers' everyday words and life experiences and specific font type and size while incorporating significant white space and concrete images that support the content it is situated with (2019). This approach significantly differs from the existing Plain Language approach. However, as there is a lack of consensus on what constitutes an acceptable level of accessible information, there is also currently no universally accepted definition for Easy English.

While each format falls under accessible information, they vary greatly in terms of accessibility, with the Plain Language being the least accessible content and Easy English being the most accessible (Basterfield, 2019, p. 16). Plain Language is currently the standard accessible information format that the Australian Government uses. However, Plain Language assumes the reader has a reading and comprehension capacity of up to ISCED level 3, which is associated with medium education. The Australian Government's preference for Plain Language as the primary accessible format overlooks that 44% of Australian adults have literacy levels between ISCED levels 0 and 2, associated with low education (Australian Bureau of Statistics, 2013).

Chinn and Buell discuss the Equality Act 2010 in the United Kingdom as a legal instrument which determines that public services make 'reasonable adjustments', including accessible information, and highlight the interpretive nature of what constitutes reasonable (Chinn & Buell, 2021, p. 629). Various standards and definitions have emerged globally from different regions or organizations. These guidelines often conflict with one another and may lack comprehensive justification for their variations (Mander, 2015). For example, UK Easy Read tends to be written for people with intellectual disabilities; however, research by Buell found that the spectrum of accessibility was widely variable and could require up to ISCED level 5 literacy (2020). This outcome highlights the problematic lack of predictability with Easy Read and is indicative of the lack of predictability within any format of accessible information.

Although beneficial to an extent, existing readability tools, such as the Flesh-Kincaid Reading Ease or the Coleman-Liau Index, cannot provide the qualitative data required to establish the basis for the standardisation of AI (Mac et al., 2022). This highlights the opportunity for investigative research into evidence-based ways to develop tools to assist the everyday person in ensuring their content is accessible to their audience.

Summary and recommendations for future policy and research directions

The policy issue of information deprivation is widespread and responsible for the exclusion of autonomous social participation of people who experience low literacy. It is also an issue that can be amended through the application and dissemination of an AI format designed to be accessible to the greatest number of people. This is achievable by employing a standardised AI format for those whose literacy abilities fall within the ISCED 0–2 level. Even with the current AI formats, the lack of consistency surrounding standards means accessibility continues to be increasingly subjective.

My lived experience of linguistic deprivation preceded a lifetime of information deprivation. Although highly literate, my access to information often depends on others to provide alternatives to listening. While we are not in the 1980s anymore and have greater access to resources, more is needed in a society that remains disabling for those who cannot bend. For example, my education has been predominantly online for over 5 years due to better access to written materials. However, audio lectures were still available to other students a week before my transcripts could be accessed. This type of experience and inequity impeded me from active participation in tutorial discussions and the learning often derived from them. Had I been taught Auslan (not Signed English), an interpreter would have been available in all situations where information was imperative to my social participation, including situations such as those in education, healthcare, work and legal settings.

The lived experience and outcomes provided in this chapter, combined with the existing and developing theories within linguistics and critical disability spaces, demonstrate the need to integrate policies to address the issue of information deprivation. The policy recommendations are:

1. Investigative research into accessible information and information deprivation. Potential areas for further research include:
    a. The structural and systematic barriers contributing to information deprivation.
    b. The financial impact of inaccessible information practices on taxpayer-funded institutions, for example, investigating the statistical relationship between low health literacy and the incidence of preventable disease.
    c. Develop evidence-based measures to create comprehensive tools for gauging accessibility of written content beyond the existing measures, which only gauge limited features relevant to the accessibility of written information (Shedlosky-Shoemaker et et al., 2009, p. 57).
    d. Find evidence-based methods for developing accessible information to ascertain the most accessible approach to its creation.
2. Allocation of research funding to inform and establish AI best practices.
3. The incorporation of AI best practices in settings that contribute to social participation and socioeconomic wellbeing within government organisations.

In conclusion, policymakers for governments and public institutions can meaningfully address information deprivation that results from inaccessible written communications via the incorporation and action of informed AI policies. Taking an AI-informed approach to written communications will reduce negative outcomes associated with information deprivation and improve access to essential information within the health, legal and financial contexts. The existing evidence establishes that information in Easy English is accessible to more people than in Plain Language or Easy Read. Further research to better understand the key characteristics that contribute to the accessibility of Easy English will assist in the development of best practices to be applied consistently within Easy English information. Therefore, utilising Easy English as the dominant accessible information format, or its equivalent in the applicable language, will ensure that essential information becomes accessible to the greatest number of people. Adopting this approach will increase effective social participation and promote positive social outcomes for people with low literacy worldwide, inherently reducing the prevalence of information deprivation experienced by people with disabilities.

References

Alim, H. S., Rickford, J. R., & Ball, A. F. (Eds.). (2016). *Raciolinguistics: How language shapes our ideas about race*. Oxford University Press.

American Library Association. (1989). American Library Association Presidential Committee on information literacy. https://www.ala.org/acrl/publications/whitepapers/presidential

Australian Bureau of Statistics. (2013). *Programme for the International Assessment of Adult Competencies, Australia* [Data set]. https://www.abs.gov.au/statistics/people/education/programme-international-assessment-adult-competencies-australia/latest-release

Australian Federation of Disability Organisations. (2025). Social Model Of Disability. Retrieved from https://afdo.org.au/social-model-of-disability/

Basterfield, C. (2019). Plain Language, Easy English. What does it all mean. *Intellectual Disability Australasia, June*(40), 15–18.

Bone, K. M. (4 2017). Trapped behind the glass: crip theory and disability identity. *Disability & Society, 32*(9), 1297–1314.

Bourdieu, P. (1991). *Language and Symbolic Power.* Harvard University Press.

Bryan, K. C., & Herrera, L. J. P. (2023). *The Weaponizing of Language in the Classroom and Beyond*. Walter de Gruyter GmbH & Co KG.

Buell, S., Langdon, P. E., Pounds, G., & Bunning, K. (2020). An open randomized controlled trial of the effects of linguistic simplification and mediation on the comprehension of 'easy read' text by people with intellectual disabilities. *Journal of Applied Research in Intellectual Disabilities: JARID, 33*(2), 219–231.

Chinn, D., & Buell, S. (2021). Easy Language in the UK. *Handbook of Easy Languages in Europe*, 623.

Commonwealth of Australia (CoA). (2023). *Royal Commission into Violence, Abuse, Neglect and Exploitation of People with Disability: Final Report: Volume 6, Enabling Autonomy and Access.* https://disability.royalcommission.gov.au/publications/final-report

Council for Intellectual Disability. (2023). Accessible information and communications - Disability Royal Commission Final Report. Retrieved from https://cid.org.au/our-stories/accessible-information/

Digital Transformation Agency. (2021). *Style Manual.* https://www.stylemanual.gov.au/content-types/easy-read

Fairclough, N. (1989). *Language and Power*. Longman.

Foucault, M. (1998). *The History of Sexuality: The Will to Knowledge.* Penguin.

Garcia, S. F., Hahn, E. A., & Jacobs, E. A. (2010). Addressing low literacy and health literacy in clinical oncology practice. *The Journal of supportive oncology*, *8*(2), 64.

Hall, M. C. (2019). Critical Disability Theory. In E. N. Zalta (Ed.), *The Stanford Encyclopedia of Philosophy* (Winter 2019). Metaphysics Research Lab, Stanford University. https://plato.stanford.edu/archives/win2019/entries/disability-critical/

Hansen-Schirra, S., & Maaß, C. (2020). Easy Language, Plain Language, Easy Language Plus: Perspectives on Comprehensibility and Stigmatisation. *Easy Language Research: Text and User Perspectives*, *2*, 17.

Henner, J., & Robinson, O. (2023). Crip linguistics goes to school. *Languages*, *8*(1), 48.

Henner, J., & Robinson, O. (2023a). Unsettling Languages, Unruly Bodyminds: A Crip Linguistics Manifesto. *Journal of Critical Study of Communication and Disability*, *1*(1), 7–37. https://doi.org/10.48516/jcscd\{_

Humphrey, J. H., & Alcorn, B. J. (1995). *So You Want to be an Interpreter?: An Introduction to Sign Language Interpreting.* H & H Publishers.

Hurtado, B., Jones, L., & Burniston, F. (2014). Is Easy Read information really easier to read? *Journal of Intellectual Disability Research: JIDR*, *58*(9), 822–829.

Jenks, A. B. (1 2019). Crip theory and the disabled identity: why disability politics needs impairment. *Disability & Society*, *34*(3), 449–469.

Kafer, A. (2013). *Feminist, Queer, Crip* (25–46). Indiana University Press.

Karlsson, M. M., & Rydström, J. (2 2023). CRIP Theory: a useful tool for social analysis. *NORA*, *31*(4), 395–410.

Kusters, A. (2021). Introduction: the semiotic repertoire: assemblages and evaluation of resources. *International Journal of Multilingualism*, *18*(2), 183–189.

Kusters, A., & Lucas, C. (2022). Emergence and evolutions: Introducing sign language sociolinguistics. *Journal of Sociolinguistics*, *26*(1), 84–98.

Mac, O., Ayre, J., Bell, K., McCaffery, K., & Muscat, D. M. (2022). Comparison of readability scores for written health information across formulas using automated vs manual measures. *JAMA Network Open*, *5*(12), e2246051.

Mander, C. (4 2015). First-hand experience of accessible information. *Tizard Learning Disability Review*, *20*(2), 80–87.

Mathews, E. S. (2017). *Language, Power, and Resistance: Mainstreaming Deaf Education*. Gallaudet University Press.

Matveeva, N., Moosally, M., & Willerton, R. (2017). Plain Language in the Twenty-First Century: Introduction to the Special Issue on Plain Language. *IEEE Transactions on Professional Communication*, *60*(4), 336–342.

McRuer, R. (6 2006). *Crip theory*. NYU Press.

Meltzer, A. (2020). Public health crises and the need for accessible information. *The Medical Journal of Australia*, *213*(10), 478–478.e1.

Morris, M. (2016). Standard White: Dismantling White normativity. *California Law Review*, *104*(4), 949.

National Deaf Children's Society. (2025). Sign language and sign systems. Retrived from https://www.ndcs.org.uk/information-and-support/language-and-communication/sign-language/what-is-a-sign-system/

NHS England. (2015). Accessible information implementation plan. *Leeds: NHS England.*

OECD. (2000). *Literacy in the Information Age Final Report of the International Adult Literacy Survey: Final Report of the International Adult Literacy Survey*. OECD Publishing.

Payne, A., Proctor, H., & Spandagou, I. (2022). The hope and burden of early intervention: Parents' educational planning for their deaf children in post-1960s Australia. *History of Education Review*, *52*(1), 69–83.

Phillipson, R. (2012). *Imperialism and colonialism* (203–235). Cambridge University Press.

Plain Language Association. (2025). What is plain language? Retrieved from https://plainlanguagenetwork.org/plain-language/what-is-plain-language/

Scope. (2015). *Clear Written Communications - The Easy English Style Guide*.

Scott, J. A., & Henner, J. (2021). Second verse, same as the first: On the use of signing systems in modern interventions for deaf and hard of hearing children in the USA. *Deafness & Education International*, *23*(2), 123–141.

Shedlosky-Shoemaker, R., Sturm, A. C., Saleem, M., & Kelly, K. M. (2009). Tools for Assessing Readability and Quality of Health-Related Web Sites. *Journal of Genetic Counselling*, *18*(1), 49–59.

Shildrick, M. (2012). 'Critical Disability Studies: rethinking the conventions for the age of postmodernity'. In *Routledge Handbook of Disability Studies*. unknown.

Skutnabb-Kangas, T. (1986). Multilingualism and the Education of Minority Children. In R. Phillipson & T. Skutnabb-Kangas (Eds.), *Linguicism Rules in Education, Parts 1–3* (42–72). Roskilde University.

Thomson, R. G. (1997). *Extraordinary Bodies: Figuring Physical Disability in American Culture and Literature*. Columbia University Press.

Townsley, R., Rodgers, J., & Folkes, L. (2003). Getting Informed: Researching the Production of Accessible Information for People with Learning Disabilities. *International Journal of Integrated Care, 11*(3), 39–43.

UNESCO. (2012). *International standard classification of education (ISCED) 2011*. UNESCO.

UNESCO Institute of Statistics. (2017). Literacy rates continue to rise from one generation to the next. *UIS Fact Sheet No.* 45

United Nations. (2006). Convention on the Rights of Persons with Disabilities. Treaty Series, 2515, 3.

Willerton, R. (2015). *Plain language and ethical action: A dialogic approach to technical content in the 21st century*. Routledge.

5

Epistemic gaps and policy absences: The plight of older people living with dual sensory impairment

Annmaree Watharow, Georgia Fagan and Moira Dunsmore

Introduction

The way we build knowledge, understand needs and create policies and services for older people living with dual sensory impairment (DSI) has to change. Article 1 of the Declaration of Human Rights states that 'all persons are born free and equal in dignity and rights' (UN, 1948). Further, the UNCRPD (UN, 2006) enshrines the right to access health and social care for all persons, irrespective of disability or difference. These conventions embed the right to protections and policies that support those living with disability, potentially allowing them to flourish at all life stages. However, for persons living with deafblindness or DSI, these protections and policies may prove inadequate due to the absence of a unique and distinct disability status in most jurisdictions. Also, a lack of visibility in society, poor data and the scarcity of lived experience accounts (Jaiswal et al., 2018) are impediments to equitable access to health and social care. So, our knowledge of those living with DSI is flawed and incomplete; these gaps, in turn, impact our policies. Failures of our knowledge production and elicitation processes create and perpetuate a lack of visibility and an absence of policies for older people living with DSI. They are fuelled, in part, by ageism, stigma and ableism. A lack of awareness of how the combination of hearing and vision loss impacts most domains of daily and social life means that those living with the losses believe them to be normal processes of ageing. There is a stigma associated with sensory loss/es that impacts disclosure and help-seeking (Dunsmore, 2022). The end self-fulfilling result is a gap in policies addressing the significant needs of this growing group and their families and carers.

Miranda Fricker's (2007) account of epistemic injustices is used in this chapter to understand the lived experience of older persons with DSI and examine how the failure of the Australian Government and institutions to recognise these has devastating consequences. We have a global challenge, too (WFDB, 2018; 2023), so the failure to account for and acknowledge lived experiences means that DSI-aware policies to deliver support and resources are absent. Also, without attention to these gaps, existing services, already so inadequate, are about to be overwhelmed as the population continues to rapidly age.

Two Australian Royal Commissions into Aged Care Quality and Safety (2021) and into Violence, Abuse, Neglect and Exploitation of People with Disability (Commonwealth of Australia, 2023) have found that the absence of policy, and therefore support, have been harmful to older people with disability. Ageism has rendered the lived experiences of older people with DSI largely invisible to Australian policymakers. Perhaps the lack of a common identity – including the absence of a society or peak body solely for older people who 'don't see too well or hear too good' – means that DSI and older age is not on the policy, protections and professional agenda.

The above-mentioned Australian Royal Commissions have also confirmed that the absence of voices of people with disability, and those of older people more generally, has contributed to the policy and service shortfalls and abuses. The voices of older people with disability are particularly absent in protections, policies, practices and research. This absence of lived experience voices – while being noted generally – is particularly evident for populations with DSI as Jaiswal et al. (2018) have noted in their literature review. Also affirming the lack of inclusion of older people with DSI broadly in protections, policies and practices is Wittich and Simcock's article, which asks: are older people with deafblindness being left behind in these arenas? (2019). We (and they) answer yes. We contend these gaps and absences are significant epistemic injustices. This chapter aims to contribute to the scant literature applying concepts of epistemic injustice and lived experience insights to ageing with DSI and discuss the implications for policy and research.

If we look specifically at older people with sensory impairment, we acknowledge that globally, they are less visible, denied basic human rights and are positioned as passive and powerless in health and social care. The World Health Organization (WHO) global priority areas include hearing loss, low vision, rapidly ageing population and loneliness (World Health Organization, 2019; World Health Organization, 2021; World Health Organization, 2023; World Health Organization, 2023a). These all converge in one population group: older adults with DSI. In Australia (as noted earlier), policies that address the specific consequences of living with DSI are absent. In this chapter, we examine the reasons for the policy shortfalls that impact this growing marginalised group. We examine the unique and distinct condition of co-occurring hearing loss and low vision through its definition, context, data and heterogeneity. Then we uncover the impacts of DSI on the individual before gazing upon national and international policy shortfalls and absences. We discuss the framing of epistemic justice, injustice and types of epistemic injustice. We look at how older people with DSI are left out of research and policy and show that this makes life for them riskier and isolated. Finally, we look at the 'hermeneutical wasteland' and blueprint on how we might move beyond the status quo of epistemic gaps and policy absences for older people with DSI.

Definition, context and heterogeneity

First, we need to understand what is DSI, or deafblindness as it is also known. Then we must contextualise ageing with sensory losses to understand why there is an urgent and growing need to address the epistemic gaps and policy absences.

Definition

DSI, deafblindness, dual sensory loss are all common terminologies that describe the combination of hearing and vision loss or impairment such that one sense cannot compensate for the other. Many older people simply say, they 'don't see too good or hear too well'. They don't get diagnosed, recognise or identify themselves as part of this group. Regardless of the presence – or absence – of terminology, recognition and identity, DSI is a unique and distinct disability (WFDB, 2018).

We use the Nordic definition and the accompanying explanatory notes which we summarise as:

> Deafblindness is a distinct disability. Deafblindness is a combined vision and hearing disability. It limits activities of a person and restricts full participation in society to such a degree that society is required to facilitate specific services, environmental alterations and/or technology.
> Nordic Welfare Centre, 2024

This definition has accompanying explanatory notes. In brief, the key complexities of life with DSI as drawn from the explanatory notes are:

1. Distinct and complex disability
2. Hard for each sense to compensate for the other
3. Time consuming
4. Energy draining
5. Information received in fragments
6. Activity limited
7. Participation reduced

8. Communication, access to information and mobility affected
9. Tactile sense critical as a conduit of information
10. Communication technology, assistive devices, interpreters and adaptations to the environment may be required
11. Despite the above, human assistance and support needed to provide access to information, mobility and safety
12. And that society is responsible for all support

Context – Defining the policy issues around DSI and older people

What do we know about older people with DSI that might explain its obscured existence in Australian health and social care policies? Primarily, there is an attenuated knowledge platform on DSI generally in Australia and other countries, plus an even thinner knowledge base on older people with DSI. Despite its impacts on health and well-being, DSI remains under-recognised in policy, practice and service delivery (Lin, 2004; WFDB, 2023). Much of the research is missing lived experience voices, delimiting our knowledge about what older people with DSI want and what they need. With a rapidly ageing population, this lack of knowledge (and data) leaves society vastly underprepared, and older citizens profoundly under-recognised and significantly under-supported.

Data

DSI prevalence globally across all age groups is estimated between 0.2% and 2%, with the majority of cases in older people

(WFDB, 2018). Since DSI is not considered a unique and distinct disability by most countries, global data collection is also inadequate. These data shortfalls limit our understanding of DSI as a global disability. The available data in Australia is deficient: we know underdiagnosis, under-reporting and inaccessibility of forms means we are constantly undercounting people with DSI. The ageing population is evident in a data shift that shows 4:1000 incidence in 2013 (Dyke, 2013) and a rate of 8:1000 by 2018 (Australian Bureaus of Statistics [ABS, 2018]). This data means that at least 200,000 Australians live with DSI, most over the age of 65 years (Australian Institute of Health and Welfare, 2019a). We are waiting on the ABS Survey of Disability Aging and Carers (SDAC) data from 2022, set for release in July 2024, which may give a clearer view.

Schneider et al. (2012) noted that prevalence of DSI increased significantly with very old age to over one in four in those aged >80 years, a trajectory confirmed by Canadian longitudinal study data (Mick et al., 2021). But there is significant data invisibility around sensory loss/es due to hidden populations, including First Nations people, residents of aged care facilities, prisoners, homeless, those with other disability and comorbidities. Misattribution is common; for example, one impairment can be conflated with another such as hearing loss with cognitive decline, or the other condition such as intoxication when a person with low vision has difficulty mobilising safely. Note that there is also premature ageing for some of these populations where the difficulties of ageing start 15 years earlier; this includes early onset sensory loss/es. For example, Australian data indicate 66% of people over 60 years have hearing loss (House of Representatives Standing

Committee on Health, Aged Care and Sport, 2017) and 6.5% of those 50 years or older have visual impairment (Foreman et al., 2016). However, among the Indigenous population, 82% of those 55 years or older have hearing loss (Australian Institute of Health and Welfare [AIHW, 2023]) and 13.6% of those over 40 years have visual impairment (AIHW, 2019), indicating both hearing and visual impairment present at higher rates and earlier onset. These 'invisible' populations mean the problem of DSI is far wider than available data suggests.

Heterogeneity

Heterogeneity is vast with diversity in age and order of onset, causation, categorisation and severity. Individuals have different resources and may have additional disability and comorbidities that complicate function and capacity.

There are six categories of older age adults with DSI, representing those ageing with DSI as well as those ageing into DSI (Wittich & Simcock, 2019; Watharow & Dunsmore, 2024). These categories are:

1. Congenitally deafblind (both hearing loss and vision loss present from birth or an early prelingual age).
2. Congenital hearing loss (non-signer) with acquired vision loss.
3. Congenital hearing loss (signer) with acquired vison loss, meaning that the principal mode of communication is compromised. This adds a cultural and linguistic diversity intersection.
4. Congenital vision loss with acquired hearing loss.
5. Acquired hearing and vision loss (this is the largest category). Causation here are common age-related conditions

such as age-related macular degeneration, cataract, glaucoma and presbycusis (age-related hearing changes) (Schneider et al., 2012).

6. Premature ageing conditions such as the rare Huntingdon-Gilford progeric syndromes (Lamis, 2022), or the more common early ageing associated with intersectional and social disadvantage (mentioned earlier).

The above categorisations rely on individuals 'knowing' they have DSI. However, a great many fall into a category of 'not knowing' or misattributing hearing loss and low vision to old age. One older person encapsulates this in a verbatim testimony, saying:

> I can't walk into a room. I see nothing and I can't find my seat and I can't recognise people. It's really hard to listen. No, not hard to listen but to hear. I try to work it out, but none of it makes any sense, you see. I know it's just old age, but I'm finding it all difficult.
> Louk, 2023

You can only be counted in data if you understand your situation, have a diagnosis or label and are asked about your sight and hearing in accessible ways. Older people with DSI can find it challenging to describe and define their sensory impairment, often viewing the losses separately (Dunsmore, 2022). This can hamper recognition of their DSI condition and diminish understanding and articulation of the complex and synergistic consequences brought on by the combined impairment. Watharow (2021) noted, 'Paradoxically, I am deafer now that I am blind. Diminution of visual cues and the impossibility of lip reading what cannot be seen increases my confusion in communication encounters' (p. 172).

There is wide heterogeneity in the severity of DSI, with combinations ranging from mild to complete sensory loss in either or both senses. Most have some residual hearing and/or vision which may be harnessed with accessibility technology, for example, hearing aid or low vison aids. Diagnostic metrics don't necessarily correspond to individual function and capacity as someone who has lived a long time with a sensory loss/es may have strategies and adjustments that someone who is newly sensory deprived in older age may not (Lee & Ottowitz, 2020). Further complicating any assessment of 'severity' and function in older adults is the high rate of multiple disability and co-occurring conditions which can be as high as 75% (WFDB, 2018). How an individual functions with their sensory loss/es depends on so many factors (as alluded to above).

Impacts of DSI

The World Federation of the Deafblind positions DSI as a complex condition that has a major influence on health and well-being of individuals, families and carers (2018). These include:

- Increased risk of functional decline as one sense cannot compensate for the other (Davidson & Guthrie, 2019).
- Impairment to an ability to complete activities of daily living and more complex instrumental activities of daily living (Brennan & Bally, 2007; Brennan et al., 2005; Guthrie et al., 2018; Heine & Browning, 2015). These complexities, in turn, potentially reduce a person's ability to age-in-place.
- Risk of social disengagement and increased dependency (Hajek & König, 2020; Jaiswal et al., 2018, 2020; Viljanen et al., 2013).
- Increased falls (Takekawa et al., 2024).

- Increased delirium (Morandi et al., 2019), visual hallucinations (Pang, 2015).
- Increased incidence of anxiety and/or depression (Bodsworth et al., 2011).
- Reduced access to healthcare (Dunsmore, 2022).
- Poor hospital experiences (Watharow, 2024; Takahashi, 2019).
- Limited access to services, information and social support that are DSI aware (Takahashi, 2019).
- 'Left behind' in disaster responses (Takayama et al., 2022).
- A complex relationship with cognitive decline (Maharani et al., 2020) and increased morbidity and mortality (Gopinath et al., 2013).
- For society, there are increased health and social care costs: age-related sensory (hearing and vision) loss is a significant health cost in Australia (AIHW, 2021) and in the United States (Huddle et al., 2016).

Policy shortfalls and absences to support older people with DSI

It is useful to define what we mean by policies. We use the WHO ICF (International Classification of Functioning, Disability and Health) terminology and definitions (World Health Organization, 2021a, p. 200); or WHO Family of International Classifications Foundation browser (World Health Organization, n.d.).

> Policies constituted by rules, regulations, conventions, and standards established by governments at the local, regional, national, and international levels, or by other recognized authorities. Policies govern and regulate the systems that organize, control, and monitor services,

structured programmes, and operations in various sectors of society.

Then this means that policies are integral to the identification of social and healthcare needs and the services that deliver necessary supports for older people with DSI.

International

International policies on ageing often fail to fully account for the unique complexities of ageing with a single sensory impairment (SSI) or DSI. These include the WHO Public health framework and Integrated Care for Older People (ICOPE). An international group are proposing a new framework for ageing with sensory loss to redress these deficiencies and accommodate the adjustments people with sensory loss can make that alters the starting points and trajectories of ageing as seen in these policy frameworks (Xiong et al., 2024; Witich et al., 2024). Another significant international policy and practice gaps has been the absence of a distinct core set of parameters for deafblindness-DSI within the WHO ICF (Billiet et al., 2021; Moeller, 2003). A core set 'facilitates the description of functioning by providing lists of essential categories that are relevant for specific health conditions and healthcare contexts'. This lack of recognition and inclusion of deafblindenss in a landmark health and rehabilitation policy framing means that the complexities and priorities around diversity in sensory function and residuals, psycho-emotional health needs and the barriers people with combined hearing and vision loss face are not accounted for in assessments and support provisions. It is as if people with DSI generally are invisible. Work is beginning on developing a tailored ICF Core Set for deafblindness; this policy and practice iteration will result in more targeted healthcare, rehabilitation and support services that actually address the needs of people with DSI (Wittich et al., 2024).

Only one-third of countries have protections and policies that recognize deafblindness-DSI as a unique and distinct disability (WFDB, 2018). In England, for example, the Care Act (2014) regulations stated that there's a requirement for specialist expertise for individuals with DSI: 6.(1) – an assessment which relates to an individual who is deafblind must be carried out by a person who has specific training and expertise relating to individuals who are deafblind.

There is currently no Australian correlation with the England Care Act but there is within the European Union (EU). In the EU, the Declaration on the rights of deafblind people (2004) states that 'deafblindness is a distinct disability of combined sight and hearing loss such that access to information, communication and orientation mobility are compromised'. Deafblind individuals therefore 'need specific support provided by people with specialist knowledge' (European Parliament, 2004).

These legislative directives have meant that protections, policies and practices attuned to the specific needs of those with DSI, including older people, are created and enacted. Member countries are required to have dedicated supports and ensure that support personnel are credentialled with specific skills to address the complexities of living with DSI.

National

Australia doesn't yet recognise DSI or deafblindness as a unique and distinct disability. It has taken several years of advocacy to the

National Disability Insurance Scheme (NDIS) to get their assessments to include deafblindness or DSI. Author one was made to 'choose' which disability was the first disability – deafness or blindness – as there was no drop-down box for DSI or deafblindness until 2024. DSI for older people is situated at the intersection of disability and ageing. In Australia, the aged care and disability governmental policymakers fail to generate distinct recognition and policies. This, in turn, means funding, services and supports are missing. People with DSI may be served by single sense services that aren't funded or aware of the complex needs of the combination. Dammeyer (2015) calls this '1 + 1 = 3', meaning that the impact is multiplicative, not additive.

There is a general lack of lived experience voices from younger and older Australians with DSI. This is highlighted by the recent defunding by the Department of Social Services, of Deafblind Australia, the peak advocacy body for people with hearing and vision loss through all life stages. This further delimits the voices calling for inclusion in policy codesign and implementation. Older people are often excluded from policies and supports for younger people, such as the NDIS where people over the age of 65 at entry cannot apply for support. In a recent review 'Getting the NDIS Bill back on track' stakeholders' feedback, strategies for older people with disability (including DSI) are conspicuously absent from proposals (AFDO, 2024). This highlights the need for the voices of older people with disability, including DSI, in the advocacy and policymaking spaces. The need for sustained, permanent funding of peak bodies with DSI lived experience representatives is a prerequisite to ensure no policymaking 'without us'.

The Royal Commission into Aged Care and Safety condemned the decades-long lack of investment by Government and found older people underserved, often unsafe with substandard systems of care (2021). We contend that policies (and knowledge, data and testimony of lived experience) are lacking in Australia to identify and meet the needs of older adults with DSI. The absence of policies perpetuates the lack of visibility and knowledge of marginalised and often hidden groups living with DSI. This absence of voices from those with DSI to inform policies and practices is a breach of epistemic or knowledge building justice.

Epistemic justice, injustice and types of epistemic injustice

Our framework for this chapter is based on Fricker's work *Epistemic Injustice: Power and the Ethics of Knowing* (Fricker, 2007). Additionally, we acknowledge that we cannot have true knowledge building justice if we aren't eliciting lived experiences in socially just ways. This means intentionally seeking out older people to relate their stories and experiences. This also means providing accessibility support and access to information alongside valuing these experiential outputs. In turn, this means providing the budgets for the increased time needed to gain the insights that will inform research and drive policy creation and iteration. This knowledge is discoverable in the experiences of marginalised individuals.

In Australia, Roy et al. (2018, p. 71) noted, 'here is a paucity of research and guidance on good practice for engaging with people who are Deafblind in policy development and the codesign of services and service systems'. They further stated that reducing power disparities, understanding sameness and diversity and deploying specialist knowledge is imperative, but including the voices of lived experience with sensory losses is non-negotiable in **all** research and policy development (Roy et al., 2018, p. 71.)

Epistemic justice

People are experts on their own lived experience, and so can identify and state what is needed, what works and what doesn't in order for social justice measures to have power. In this way, knowledge building, that is, epistemology, is inextricably linked to social justice and inclusion. Epistemic insights are also essential to determining if our social and health institutions are indeed providing the services the community requires and of a quality that the community expects.

Truly inclusive knowledge building practices must aim to tackle the current inherent epistemic injustices. If data collection methods exclude certain populations, this data will perpetuate forms of epistemic injustices through its silencing of particular perspectives.

Epistemic injustice

'Epistemic injustice' refers to Fricker's concept of the wrong done to somebody in their capacity as a holder of knowledge and includes both hermeneutical and testimonial injustice (Fricker, 2007, p. 1). Epistemic injustice occurs when the seekers of knowledge fail to locate and make legible the testimonies of the historically marginalised by discriminating, devaluing, ignoring or erasing the knowledge that is held by these knowers. Fricker's framing positions the knower as the centre of knowledge, and any failure to seek, value and make visible this knowledge constitutes an epistemic injustice being done to that knower. Data identification, collection and evaluation methods that are used to inform policies in disability older care, in their current forms exclude, wrongly interpret or fail to reach the intended people. Researchers can devalue and dismiss testimonies of marginalised groups and individuals, based on ableist and discriminatory attitudes and beliefs about trustworthiness. Testimonies of proxies or researcher interpretations may prevail in the place of accounts of lived experiences of disability and ageing.

Fricker's 2007 work is having a renaissance in research, especially research around disability, inclusion and the concerns of many marginalised groups. For example:

- McKinnon (2019) – gaslighting as epistemic injustice
- CohenMiller & Boivin (2021) – criminal justice system and young offenders' legal literacy
- Groot (B) (2022) – health and ethics of care
- Isham et al. (2019) – female family carer violence

Types of epistemic injustice

There are three typologies of epistemic injustices – testimonial, hermeneutical and co-occurrent. A testimonial injustice occurs when the credibility of a speaker's knowledge is undermined by the hearer due to the hearer's possession of a prejudicial stereotype about the identity of the speaker (Fricker, 2007, p. 1). In such cases, the speaker's testimony, perhaps their explication of pain or disenfranchisement, may be either distrusted or altogether ignored by the hearer due to, for example, age, gender or perceived ability of the speaker.

An older person's testimony is often regarded as less believable and less competent. Health and social carers and researchers create judgements about credibility, irrespective of older adults' capacity or actual ability. Ageism is commonplace and discriminatory stereotyping alongside ageist attitudes further marginalises older people and their lived experiences (Allen et al., 2022).

Hermeneutical injustices occur when an individual or group of individuals are unable to render their experiences intelligible to either themselves or others due to the existence of systemic prejudices (or lacunas) in the collective hermeneutical resources (Fricker 2007, p. 154). This may be due to a lack of appropriate terminology or because of the individual's context denying them insight as to the existence of such terminology. Fricker's original example explores the case of a woman experiencing workplace sexual harassment prior to the creation of the concept 'sexual harassment'. In such a case, this woman is unable to employ this term as a means to render her experience intelligible to both her and others.

In the case of older people living with DSI, instances of testimonial and hermeneutical injustices can and mostly do co-occur in myriad ways. A testimonial injustice occurs, for example, when the epistemic insights of those living with DSI are inadequately sought and received in healthcare research settings (Watharow et al., 2024). Systemic, hermeneutical injustices occur among this population due to prejudices in the collective hermeneutical resources such as contemporary health policies, which diminish or altogether neglect the harms and difficulties faced by those ageing with and into DSI. Without this and other forms of sufficient recognition, people with DSI are unable to achieve the self and collective acknowledgement necessary to resolve their susceptibility to different types of injustice (Fricker, 2007, p. 156).

The rise and perpetuation of epistemic wrongs

When considering the epistemic wrongs done to older people living with DSI by policy absences, we need to examine the role of testimonial and hermeneutical injustices. They are concurrent in the DSI group. The prejudices and stereotypes exist alongside the lack of hermeneutical resources for older people to navigate what is going on, within them as well as around them.

This lack of awareness of their sensory losses being more than 'just old age' means that there is no identity with a condition nor a knowledge of the supports available. These hermeneutical lacunae are not limited to individuals, but also extend to a lack of awareness, insight and interest from community, health and social care institutions, policymakers and governments.

Accessibility and epistemic insights

Accessibility and its role in epistemic justice

In the pursuit of epistemic insights to inform protections, policies and research, the role of accessibility cannot be overstated. There is a lack of research specifically around best practice for accessibility provision in older people with DSI. Roy et al.'s work centres around deafblind adults primarily under 65 years (2018). Lack of accessibility provisions and a disregard for the funds and time needed to gain insights perpetuates testimonial and hermeneutical injustices. We use Tichkosky's (2011) definition of accessibility as a 'complex form of perception that organises socio-political relations between people in social space' (p. 9). If accessibility is provided, power imbalance is mitigated; if it's not provided, then the knower is silenced or ignored by the more powerful. This perpetuates knowledge gaps and allows inadequate or unsafe systems to continue to flourish. The role of accessibility provision in promoting epistemic justice has been little explored, although it is alluded to in the final chapter of Fricker's 2007 work. Fricker explains how differences in form and style of language and communication can contribute to hermeneutical injustices with voices being stifled or remaining silent.

Fricker writes, 17 years after her seminal book, more explicitly that failure to provide accessibility points to 'the distinctive intelligibility disadvantage experienced by those who speak, write, and sign differently from what is expected/habitual in the context provided' (Personal communication via email, Fricker, 10 November, 2023). Older people with sensory losses may therefore be hermeneutically marginalised by their needs for more time for communication exchanges, different lighting, alternate formats, assistive technology and face-to-face preferences. Fricker elaborates:

> Belonging to a group whose expressive style (perhaps a distinctive way of signing, for instance) can be a form of hermeneutical marginalisation. And so, when that style is not sufficiently shared with those to whom one is hoping to communicate, that can result in an unfair deficit of intelligibility—a hermeneutical injustice.

Personal communication via email, Fricker 10 November, 2023

Researchers, policymakers and service providers are therefore required to intentionally prioritise accessibility (and the funds and time needed). Older people who don't see too well or hear too good cannot compensate for one diminished sense by using the other. This means that for each individual, ways need to be explored that promote their access to information and ability to communicate their experiences and requisites. Without this intentionality and resourcing, hermeneutical injustices are perpetuated, data remains scant, policies inadequate and social institutions fail to meet community expectations.

Being seen, heard and included depends on being able to view the online surveys, hear the researchers' questions and notice their lips and facial cues, navigate the online platform and understand what is being said, for example, in noisy focus groups. Giving informed consent may require a large print document or an explanation in a quiet room. For some, braille materials or tactile language support by interpreters are needed. Accessibility is not simply about technology and devices but relational: how we ask what is needed and how we provide that for each individual is key. How we recognise that we need to consider our own presentation and actions (Do we have an accent? Speak too quickly? Ask questions and give information while facing a laptop and not the person in front of us? to name a few). In lived experience-led DSI work, negotiation as to which communication mode suits everyone in the conversation best is necessary (e.g. Watharow & Mellifont, 2024). This should be a normalised practice where knowledge seekers and the expert knowers acquire an understanding of – and accommodate – one another's specific communication and support needs.

The importance of epistemic insights

This chapter establishes that older people with DSI are the expert knowers of their own conditions, circumstances and experiences, even if these are not nameable, sought, counted or valued. When the testimonies of particular individuals and communities are unsought, unheard or silenced, a wrong is done to both the expert knower and to the communities that would have benefited from their knowledge. In order to know and serve our society and its communities (including institutions, policies and services), we, researchers, policymakers, service providers and health and social care institutions must ensure that we construct knowledge with those knowers experiencing the individual institution's research, policies and services (or lack thereof). Evaluating the performance of community systems designed to serve older people with DSI depends on direct testimony from those older individuals. As the Australian Royal Commission highlighted, the absence of lived experience knowledge informing and evaluating the social institutions and policies supposed to serve them are decades-long systemic failures that result in parlous states of care and actual harm for older adults, especially those living with disability. A wrong is also committed against broader society as its institutions, policies and systems remain unchecked, inefficient and uninformed by the perpetuation of not only epistemic injustices but exclusion from social life and shared decision-making in healthcare, for example.

Epistemic insights are vital in another capacity; the more lived experiences are heard and seen, the greater the community recognition of the existence of DSI as a distinct condition. Its complexities and challenges need not be endured without support. The stigma and ageism will be challenged. The greater that community awareness, the greater the epistemic power that can voice demand for policy recognition and redress. Fricker's earlier example about sexual harassment illustrates this.

These gaps in epistemic insights represent lost opportunities to change the status quo, improving quality of life in those ageing with and into DSI and so also reducing health and social care costs. Huddle et al. (2016) and others have shown that better management of SSI and DSI would be fiscally efficient.

The wasteland and what lies beyond

The hermeneutical wasteland

A hermeneutical lack of awareness centres around how sensory loss/es are not simply 'unavoidable, un-remediable part of ageing'. Those living with DSI are invisible, their invisibility made endemic by the limited individual, community and professional knowledge about DSI. This ignorance diminishes an individual's ability to develop an understanding of their circumstances and access to services and support. Without this awareness, those in need do not realise the possibilities for reducing their isolation and their challenges, nor can they advocate for the policy assistance that can aid health and well-being.

According to Fricker, these epistemic and hermeneutical absences constitute injustices when they prevent a person from 'understanding a significant patch' of their own experiences, 'a patch of experience which it is strongly in her interests to understand, for without that understanding she is left deeply troubled, confused, and isolated, not to mention vulnerable to continued harassment' (Fricker, 2007, p. 151).

This chapter argues that those living with DSI face these injustices, in addition to the numerous harms and risks they engender. Given this, society needs to better understand how these wrongs arise and are maintained. It needs to reconfigure our collective epistemic resources into a more desirable, just forms. To build hermeneutical resources that older people with DSI and their families need – this demands a whole-of-society policy and action response. Everyone has the right to grow older as well as the possibility to access quality healthcare, enjoy life-long learning, share in decision-making and participate in all desired domains of social life. As the United Nations Secretary General (UNSDG, n.d.) remarked, 'Only by working together – across governments, international organizations, civil society, and the private sector – can we effectively implement the Convention on the Rights of Persons with Disabilities and deliver on the 2030 Agenda for Sustainable Development for persons with disabilities'.

Older people with DSI often experience hermeneutic marginalisation, exile to a wasteland, as their insights and experiences are insufficiently expressed. Without these expressions, our collective hermeneutical resources become structurally prejudiced (Fricker, 2007 p. 154), maintaining a systemic incapacity for those in need to access the epistemic resources necessary to resolve their marginalisation and injustice. As mentioned in the Introduction, older people with DSI are globally less visible and denied basic human rights. They are positioned as passive and powerless in health and social care. In Australia, policies that address the specific consequences of living with DSI are absent, so inequities and oppression continue. Moreover, while older people with DSI lack a constructive way of labelling themselves, professionals veer between the labels of deafblindness and DSI or loss (Wittich et al., 2013) while missing large numbers of individuals with the condition. Non-uniformity surrounding labelling can have debilitating impacts on the formation of robust, expedient, useful interventions. Compounding this is the more general lack of recognition by professionals who fail to acknowledge presence, significant complexities and challenges of living with DSI.

The hermeneutic wasteland is thus a cheerless, complex space beset by the demons of not knowing what is happening, feelings of shame and a wider social and health system not knowledgeable or equipped to recognise and remediate.

Leaving the wasteland

To escape the hermeneutic wasteland of growing older into and with SSI and DSI, we need to trust and access the wisdom of the expert knowers. Sensory impairments will come to all of us, one way or another, whether ourselves, parents, partner, family, friends, patients, clients, customers. The data which underestimates the incidence of sensory loss inform us that 66% of us will have hearing loss of some kind by age 60 (House of Representative Committee, 2017), and one-third of us will have some form of eye condition in older age (Foreman et al., 2017).

We need to talk about SSI and DSI now. We need to allocate resources, write policy, educate health and social care practitioners, provide services and educate communities. We need to give older people the hermeneutic resources to understand that their sensory losses are not unavoidable or unsupportable. In short, we need to advise that there are strategies and supports, information and resources, care and communication to be had. While professionals and practitioners charged with the care of older people remain unaware of DSI and its impacts on older people, they also fail to validate the complex lives of those in their care, meaning that the lived experience of those who 'don't see too good or hear too well' remains unacknowledged. The potential for harm exists in ignorance and as the Royal Commissions reveal harm has been enacted time and again.

A sense of identity and knowing DSI as a real and distinct condition is needed to help individuals and families navigate out of the wasteland. The ways which people have available to them to know that things could be different, or more specifically, could be better, are manifold as many as the individuals with DSI and their differing communication needs. These ways are dependent on recognition. The individuals, even if they can't see well and hear better, can be better supported to live a higher quality life.

In tangible ways, epistemic (in)justice is about expectations; rectifying it involves a reconsideration of expectations. Often, we accept the things we have come to expect as normal, when they are normalised. We accept taxation, for instance, because we consider taxes provide benefits. But unquestioning expectations of hearing and vision degradation as we age and a concurrent general lack of support signal that degradation is inevitable as death and taxes. This perspective benefits no one. Our task is to consider the ways of altering a status quo that perpetuates and internalises ageism, ableism, harm and neglect.

A policy and research guide to building hermeneutic resources and promoting epistemic and social justice for people with DSI

To create change in epistemically just ways is to enable a dynamic engagement between the target population with DSI and policymakers. We offer a policy and research guide for exiting these hermeneutic wastelands:

1. Recognition by government of the distinct disability status and dedicated policy and support needs of people with DSI.
2. Intentionally seeking out older people to relate their stories and experiences. There should be no knowledge creation, research or policy without lived experience insights.
3. Listening to expert knowers with lived experience of DSI and ensuring their visibility and inclusion in policymaking is key.
4. Include families and carers. Lived experience insights of all stakeholders are critical to building a strong knowledge platform.
5. All disability research and policy to be co-produced in a collective manner with lived experience insights.
6. Provide accessible ways of eliciting lived experience insights: researchers and policymakers must budget and plan for the necessary time and resources.

7. A broad investment by Government in older care for those ageing in place and in residential aged care alike.
8. Skilling, upskilling and reskilling the existing aged care workforce in the specific needs of those with sensory loss/es and their families/carers. This will require development, implementation and wide acceptance of micro credentialling.
9. Skilling, upskilling and reskilling professionals as well as practitioners. This includes students in health and social care. No one can leave the wastelands without recognition of the condition of DSI with diagnosis, discussion and referrals for supports.
10. Information provision in multiple formats and media, such as a consumer handbook for those with DSI, their families and carers. They can't leave the wastelands without a trustworthy guidebook.
11. Get the data right: use accessible methods, seek out the hidden populations and provide funding for these research endeavours.
12. Future policymaking needs to be co-produced and addressed: dedicated dual sensory support services, include families and carers as stakeholders, robust social support and raising awareness and skills at all levels.
13. Future research directions need to centre on co-production and accessible methodologies examining what people with DSI find helpful to achieve goals and improve quality of life.
14. Finally, we need lived experience-led research and policymaking: this means 'growing' and providing opportunities for people with DSI to generate and lead research and policy. This will require investment in disabled people's

organisations and providing research and policy writing skills acquisition opportunities. It will mean remunerating lived experience representatives to develop and advance as well as participate and contribute.

Conclusion

In this chapter, we explored some complexities and challenges of living with DSI for older people, families and carers. We linked epistemic injustices, both testimonial and hermeneutic, with the invisible epidemic of older people with DSI.

The keys to understanding why DSI is missing in action from policy and supports are linked in every way to a lack of epistemic insights from those living with DSI. These lacks and policy gaps result in the creation of a hermeneutic wasteland and deprives older people of resources to recognise, adjust to and manage DSI.

We have given a research and policy blueprint to promote epistemic insights and dedicated, targeted policymaking. However, essentially you can distil this discussion to one point: listen to the expert knowers, the people themselves and also to their families/carers in ways that work for them, so that any research is ethical and just, so the epistemology is truthful and the policies are codeveloped addressing the communities' needs. In this way, getting older with or acquiring sensory losses doesn't mean negative health outcomes, greater risks and being left out of social domains. In Australia, DSI-specific policies, practices and supports are missing. We contend that asking the expert knowers, that is, including lived experience and lived expertise voices in research, policy and practice, can catalyse needful change. With equitable research practices, better knowledge co-production, inclusive policymaking and greater individual, family/carer, professional and community awareness and accommodations, older people with DSI can be happier, healthier and safer.

References

Allen, J. O., Solway, E., Kirch, M., Singer, D., Kullgren, J. T., Moïse, V., & Malani, P. N. (2022). Experiences of everyday ageism and the health of older US adults. *JAMA Network Open*, *5*(6), e2217240–e2217240.

Australian Bureau of Statistics. (2018). *Survey of disability, ageing and carers, Australia: Summary of findings*. https://www.abs.gov.au/statistics/health/disability/disability-ageing-and-carers-australia-summary-findings/latest-release

Australian Federation of Disability Organisations (AFDO). (2024). – Response to final recommendations from Independent review of the National Disability Insurance Scheme (NDIS?). Retrieved 24 July from https://www.afdo.org.au/wp-content/uploads/2024/05/2024_05-AFDO-Response-to-the-NDIS-Review-Report-May-2024-Final.pdf

Australian Government, Department of Social Services, (n.d.) *Disability and Carers, National Disability Insurance Scheme.* Can I access the NDIS? Retrieved July 9, 2024, from https://www.dss.gov.au/disability-and-carers/programmes-services/for-people-with-disability/national-disability-insurance-scheme#02

Australian Institute of Health and Welfare. (2021). *Disease expenditure in Australia 2018–19.2021*. https://www.aihw.gov.au/reports/health-welfare-expenditure/disease-expenditure-australia/contents/australian-burden-of-disease-groups

Australian Institute of Health and Welfare. (2023). *Ear and hearing health of Aboriginal and Torres Strait Islander people* 2023–4 December 2023, accessed July 9, 2024 https://www.aihw.gov.au/reports/indigenous-australians/ear-hearing-health-indigenous-people-2023/summary

Australian Institute of Health and Welfare. (2019). *Homelessness and homelessness services*. https://www.aihw.gov.au/reports/australias-welfare/homelessness-and-homelessness-services

Australian Institute of Health and Welfare. (2019a). ABS Survey of Disability, Aging and Carers (SDAC), 2018, Retrived from https://meteor.aihw.gov.au/content/731625

Billiet, L., Van de Velde, D., Overbury, O., & Van Nispen, R. M. (2021). International classification of functioning, disability and health core set for vision loss: A discussion paper and invitation. *British Journal of Visual Impairment*, *40*(2), pp.109–116. https://doi.org/10.1177/02646196211055954

Bodsworth, S. M., Clare, I. C. H., & Simblett, S. K. (2011). Deafblindness and mental health: Psychological distress and unmet need among adults with dual sensory impairment. *British Journal of Visual Impairment, 29*(1), 6–26. https://doi.org/10.1177/0264619610387495

Brennan, M., and Bally, S. J. (2007). Psychosocial adaptations to dual sensory loss in middle and late adulthood. *Trends in Amplification*, *11*(4), pp. 281–300. https://doi.org/10.1177/1084713807308210

Brennan, M., Horowitz, A., & Su, Y.-P. (2005). Dual sensory loss and its impact on everyday competence. *The Gerontologist, 45*(3), pp. 337–346. https://doi.org/10.1093/geront/45.3.337

Care Act 2014, UK Public General Acts. https://www.legislation.gov.uk/ukpga/2014/23/contents, accessed July 9, 2024.

CohenMiller, A. and Boivin, N. (2021). *Questions in qualitative social justice research in multicultural contexts* (1st ed.). Routledge.

Commonwealth of Australia. (2023). *Royal Commission into Violence, Abuse, Neglect and Exploitation of People with Disability: Final Report*. Available from: https://www.royalcommission.gov.au/publications/final-report

Davidson, J. G. S., & Guthrie, D. M. (2019). Older adults with a combination of vision and hearing impairment experience higher rates of cognitive impairment, functional dependence, and worse outcomes across a set of quality indicators. *Journal of Aging and Health*, *31*(1), pp. 85–108. https://doi.org/10.1177/0898264317723407

Dammeyer, J. (2015). Deafblindness and dual sensory loss research: Current status and future directions. *World Journal of Otorhinolaryngology*, *5*(2), 37–40.

Deafblind Nordic Cooperation Committee. *Nordens välfärdscenter* (Nordic Welfare Centre) (2018). *Nordic definition of deafblindness*. https://nordicwelfare.org/wp-content/uploads/2018/03/nordic-definition-of-deafblindness.pdf

Dunsmore, M. (2022). *An invisible disability: Navigating the enduring state of dual sensory impairment (DSI) in older age*, PhD thesis, Faculty of Medicine and Health, The University of Sydney, Sydney, Australia. https://hdl.handle.net/2123/29262

Dyke, P. (2013). *A clear view: Identifying Australians who live with deafblindness and dual sensory loss*. Senses Australia. https://www.senseswa.com.au/wp-content/uploads/2016/01/a-clear-view-senses-australia.pdf

European Parliament, (2004) *Declaration of the European Parliament on the rights of deafblind people, 2004*. https://www.europarl.europa.eu/doceo/document/DCL-5-2004-0001_EN.pdf

Foreman, J., Keel, S., Xie, J., van Wijngaarden, P., Crowton, J., Taylor, H.R. & Dirani, M. (2016). *The national eye health survey 2016*, Vision 2020 Australia, Melbourne, viewed 12 October 2017, https://www.vision2020australia.org.au/wp-content/uploads/2019/06/National-Eye-Health-Survey_Full-Report_FINAL.pdf.

Foreman, J., Xie, J., Keel, S., van Wijngaarden, P., Sandhu, S. S., Ang, G. S., Fan Gaskin, J., Crowston, J., Bourne, R., Taylor, H. R., & Dirani, M. (2017). The prevalence and causes of vision loss in Indigenous and non-Indigenous Australians: The national eye health survey.

Ophthalmology, 124(12), pp. 1743–1752. https://doi.org/10.1016/j.ophtha.2017.06.001

Fricker, M. (2023). *Epistemic injustice: Power and the ethics of knowing*, Oxford University Press.

Gopinath, B., Schneider, J., McMahon, C. M., Burlutsky, G., Leeder, S. R., & Mitchell, P. (2013). Dual sensory impairment in older adults increases the risk of mortality: A population-based study. *PLoS One, 8*(3), Article e55054. https://doi.org/10.1371/journal.pone.0055054

Groot, B., Haveman, A., & Abma, T. (2022). Relational, ethically sound co-production in mental health care research: epistemic injustice and the need for an ethics of care. *Critical Public Health, 32*(2), 230–240. https://doi.org/10.1080/09581596.2020.1770694

Guthrie, D. M., Davidson, J. G. S., Williams, N., Campos, J., Hunter, K., Mick, P., Orange, J. B., Pichora-Fuller, M. K., Phillips, N. A., Savundranayagam, M. Y., & Wittich, W. (2018). Combined impairments in vision, hearing and cognition are associated with greater levels of functional and communication difficulties than cognitive impairment alone: Analysis of interRAI data for home care and long-term care recipients in Ontario. *PloS one, 13*(2), e0192971. https://doi.org/10.1371/journal.pone.0192971

Hajek, A., & König, H-H. (2020). Dual sensory impairment and healthcare use: Findings from a nationally representative sample. *Geriatrics & Gerontology International, 20*(6), pp. 602–606. https://doi.org/10.1111/ggi.13929

Heine, C., & Browning, C. J. (2015). Dual Sensory loss in older adults: a systematic review *The Gerontologist*, Volume 55, Issue 5, October 2015, pp. 913–928, https://doi.org/10.1093/geront/gnv074

House of Representatives Standing Committee on Health, Aged Care and Sport (2017), *Still waiting to be heard … Report on the Inquiry into the Hearing Health and Wellbeing of Australia*, Parliament of the Commonwealth of Australia, Canberra, viewed14 September2017,https://parlinfo.aph.gov.au/parlInfo/download/committees/reportrep/024048/toc_pdf/Stillwaitingtobeheard....pdf;fileType=application/pdf

Huddle, M. G., Deal, J. A., Swenor, B., Genther, D. J., & Lin, F. R. (2016). Association between dual sensory impairment, hospitalization, and burden of disease. *Journal of the American Geriatrics Society*, *64*(8), pp. 1735–1737. https://doi.org/10.1111/jgs.14210

Isham, L., Bradbury-Jones, C., & Hewison, A. (2019). Female family carers' experiences of violent, abusive or harmful behaviour by the older person for whom they care: a case of epistemic injustice?. *Sociology of health & illness*, *42*(1), 80–94. https://doi.org/10.1111/1467-9566.12986

Jaiswal, A., Aldersey, H., Wittich, W., Mirza, M., & Finlayson, M. (2018). Participation experiences of people with deafblindness or dual sensory loss: A scoping review of global deafblind literature. *PLoS One, 13*(9), Article e0203772. https://doi.org/10.1371/journal.pone.0203772

Jaiswal, A., Fraser, S., & Wittich, W. (2020). Barriers and facilitators that influence social participation in older adults with dual sensory impairment. *Frontiers in Education*, *5*, Article 127. https://doi.org/10.3389/feduc.2020.00127

Lamis, A., Siddiqui, S.W., Ashok, T., Patni, N., Fatima, M., Aneef, A.N. (2022). Hutchinson-Gilford Progeria Syndrome: A Literature Review. *Cureus, 14(8)*. https://doi.org/10.7759/cureus.28629

Lee, H. & Ottowitz, J. (2020). *Foundations of Vision Rehabilitation Therapy*. APH Press, American Printing House for the Blind.

Louk, I. (Director). Watharow, A. (Writer). (2023) Dramatised verbatim testimony of DSI hospital experiences, Lucy's Story [Film; educational Vimeo private access]. Faculty of Medicine and Health, University of Sydney.

Lin, M. Y., Gutierrez. P. R., Stone, K. L., Yaffe, K., Ensrud, K., Fink, H. A., Sarkisian, C. A., Coleman, A. L., & Mangione, C. M. (2004).

Vision impairment and combined vision and hearing impairment predict cognitive and functional decline in older women. *Journal of the American Geriatrics Society, 52*(12), pp. 1996–2002. https://agsjournals.onlinelibrary.wiley.com/doi/abs/10.1111/j.1532-5415.2004.52554.x

Maharani, A., Dawes, P., Nazroo, J., Tampubolon, G., & Pendleton, N. (2020). Associations between self-reported sensory impairment and risk of cognitive decline and impairment in the Health and Retirement Study cohort. *The Journals of Gerontology. Series B, Psychological Sciences and Social Sciences, 75*(6), 1230–1242. https://doi.org/10.1093/geronb/gbz043

McKinnon, R. (2019). Gaslighting as epistemic violence: "allies", mobbing, and complex posttraumatic stress disorder, including a case study of harassment of transgender women in sport. In B. R. Sherman & S. Goguen (Eds.), *Overcoming Epistemic Injustice: Social and Psychological Perspectives*. Rowman and Littlefield International.

Mellifont, D., Watharow, A., Daniels-Mayes, S., Smith-Merry, J., O'Donovan, M-A. (2024). Ethical inclusion and participation of people with disability in research: problematising vulnerability in A. Good, I. Elliott & S. Mallon (Eds.). *Advances in Disability Research Ethics*, Emerald Publishing Limited.

Mick, P.T., Hämäläinen, A., Kolisang, L., Pichora-Fuller, M. K., Phillips, N., Gutherie, D., Wittich, W. (2021). The prevalence of hearing, vision, and dual sensory loss in older Canadians: An analysis of data from the Canadian longitudinal study on Aging. *Canadian Journal on Aging, 40*(1), pp. 1–22. https://doi.org/10.1017/S0714980820000070

Möeller, K., (2003) Deafblindness: a challenge for assessment: Is the ICF a useful tool? *International Journal of Audiology 42* (sup1), pp. 140–142.

Morandi, A., Di Santo, S. G., Zambon, A., Mazzone, A., Cherubini, A. Mossello, E., Bo, M., Marengoni, A., Bianchetti, A, Cappa, S.,

Fimognari, F., Incalzi, R. A., Gareri, P., Perticone, F., Campanini, M., Penco, I., Montorsi, M., Di Bari, M., Trabucchi, M., Bellelli, G. (2019). Italian Study Group on Delirium (ISGoD), Delirium, dementia, and In-hospital mortality: The results from the Italian Delirium Day 2016, A national multicenter study. *The Journals of Gerontology: Series A*, 74(6), pp. 910–916, https://doi.org/10.1093/gerona/gly154

Nordic Welfare Centre. (2024). Nordic definition on deafblindness. Retrieved from https://nordicwelfare.org/wp-content/uploads/2024/11/nordicdefinition-2.pdf

Pang, L. (2015). Visual hallucinations: Identifying Charles Bonnet syndrome. *International Journal of Ophthalmology & Eye Science*, pp14–22. https://doi.org/10.19070/2332-290X-SI01004

Roy, A., McVilly, K. R., Crisp, B. (2018). Preparing for inclusive consultation, research and policy development: insights from the field of Deafblindness. *Journal of Social Inclusion*, *9* (1), 71–88. https://pdfs.semanticscholar.org/5cd6/d525ef8a3b9cfe40f8e800532a48fb641391.pdf

Royal Commission into Aged Care Quality and Safety. (2021). Royal Commission into Aged Care Report *Care, Dignity and Respect 2021*, Australian Government Royal Commission into Aged Care Quality and Safety:https://nla.gov.au/nla.obj-2928215218/view, accessed July 9.

Schneider, J., G. Bamini, C McMahon, E. Teber, S.R, Leeder, J. J. Wang, P. Mitchell. (2012). Prevalence and 5-year incidence of Dual Sensory Impairment in an Older Australian Population, *Annals of Epidemiology*, *22* (4), pp. 295–301. https://www.sciencedirect.com/science/article/abs/pii/S1047279712000191

Takahashi, N. (2019). 'Accessibility for people with deafblindness when getting medical services', Deafblind International World Conference, 12–16 August, Gold Coast, Australia.

Takayama, K., Craig, L., Cooper, A., Stokar, H. (2022). Exploring deaf students' disaster awareness and preparedness in U.S. higher education settings: Implications for university-level DRR policy and programming, *International Journal of Disaster Risk Reduction,* Vol 83. https://doi.org/10.1016/j.ijdrr.2022.103409

Takekawa, T., Obuchi, K., Watanabe, S., Yamada, N., & Abo, M. (2024). A 10-Year Study of the Trend of Accidental Falls in the Elderly in a Japanese Hospital. Advance online publication. https://doi.org/10.1055/a-2276-0011

Titchkosky, T. (2011). *The question of access: Disability, space, meaning,* University of Ontario Press. https://www.researchgate.net/profile/Tanya-Titchkosky/publication/303419533_The_Question_of_Access_Disability_Space_Meaning/links/5b9a694245851574f7c3d216/The-Question-of-Access-Disability-Space-Meaning.pdf

United Nations General Assembly. (1948). *The Universal Declaration of Human Rights* (UDHR). New York: United Nations General Assembly.

United Nations General Assembly (2006). *Convention on the Rights of Persons with Disabilities (CRPD)* New York: United Nations General Assembly. Date 13 December 2006. https://www.ohchr.org/en/hrbodies/crpd/pages/conventionrightspersonswithdisabilities.aspx

United Nations Sustainable Development Group [UNSDG]. (n.d.). Advancing the rights of persons with disabilities around the world. Retrieved July 24, 2024, from https://unsdg.un.org/latest/blog/secretary-general-remarks-global-disability-summit

Viljanen, A., Törmäkangas, T., Vestergaard, S., & Andersen-Ranberg, K. (2013). Dual sensory loss and social participation in older Europeans. *European Journal of Ageing, 11*(2), pp. 155–167. https://doi.org/10.1007/s10433-013-0291-7

Watharow, A. T. (2021). *'Not knowing what is going on': The experiences of people with deafblindness–dual sensory impairment in Australian hospitals—a mixed methods study* (Doctoral dissertation).

Watharow, A. (2024). Australian Hospital Experiences of People Living with Deafblindness or Dual Sensory Impairment: The Report Card. *Healthcare* (Basel), *12*(8), 852-. https://doi.org/10.3390/healthcare12080852

Watharow, A., & Dunsmore, M. (2024). *Dual sensory impairment and the older person: A silent epidemic*, Lived Places Publishing.

Watharow, A., Joseph, S., & Fagan, G. (2024). Creating Ethical Storytelling Spaces, in Research and Beyond, for People Living with Disability and Trauma. In Rasmussen, A. J. & Sodemann, M. (Eds.) *Narrative Medicine: Trauma and Ethics* (pp. 3–14). Vernon Press.

Watharow, A., & Mellifont, D. (2024). A case study unveiling challenges and supports for deafblind and neurodivergent researchers and participants. *Journal of Humanity and Social Justice.*, 109–123.

Wittich, W., multiple other authors, (2024) article under review from *The Gerontologist*, Oxford University Press.

Wittich, W., Dumassais, S., Prain, M.m McVilly, K., Anze, D., Lopez, R., Minhas, R., van de Molengraft, S., Baur, M., Jaiswal, A., Gravel, C., Ogedengbe, T. O., Granberg, S. (2024). Perspectives from individuals living with deafblindness on priorities for the development of WHO ICF Core Sets. Presented at the ARVO Annual Meeting, Seattle, WA, May 5-9, 2024.

Wittich, W. and Simcock, P., (2019). Aging and combined vision and hearing loss. In J. Ravencroft (Ed.) *The Routledge Book of Visual Impairment*. (pp. 438–456) Routledge.

Wittich, W., Southall, K., Sikora, L., Watanabe, D. H., & Gagné, J.-P. (2013). What's in a name: Dual sensory impairment or deafblindness? *British Journal of Visual Impairment, 31*(3), 198–207. https://doi.org/10.1177/0264619613490519

World Federation of the Deafblind. (2018). At risk of exclusion from CRPD and SDGs implementation: Inequality and persons with deafblindness. Initial global report on situation and rights of persons with deafblindness. http://www.wfdb.eu/wp-content/uploads/2019/04/WFDB-global-report-2018.pdf

World Federation of the Deafblind. (2023). *WFDB Second Global Report 2023: Good Practices and Recommendations for the Inclusion of Persons with Deafblindness*. https://wfdb.eu/wfdb-report-2022/

World Health Organization. (n.d.). WHO Family of International Classifications Foundation: Browse info. Retrieved from https://icd.who.int/browse/2024-01/foundation/en#949333446

World Health Organization. (2019). Integrated care for older people (ICOPE) implementation framework: Guidance for systems and services. https://www.who.int/publications/i/item/9789241515993

World Health Organization. (2021) *World report on hearing*. https://www.who.int/teams/noncommunicable-diseases/sensory-functions-disability-and-rehabilitation/highlighting-priorities-for-ear-and-hearing-care

World Health Organization. (2021a). *International Classification of Functioning, Disability and Health*. Geneva, Switzerland.

World Health Organization. (2023) *World report on vision*. https://www.who.int/publications/i/item/9789241516570

World Health Organization. (2023a). WHO launches commission to foster social connection. https://www.who.int/news/item/15-11-2023-who-launches-commission-to-foster-social-connection (accessed Nov 2023)

Xiong, Y., Nemargut, J.P., Bradley, C., Wittich, W., Legge, G. E. (2024) Development and validation of a questionnaire for assessing visual and auditory spatial localization abilities in dual sensory impairment. *Scientific Reports 14*(7911) (2024). https://doi.org/10.1038/s41598-024-58363-6

6
Charcot-Marie-Tooth disease in rural Australia: A retrospective analysis of research and policy observation

Scott Denton

Introduction

It has been well documented that there are significant differences in healthcare service delivery between rural and metropolitan Australia which has led to inequities (National Rural Health Alliance, 2023). However, underneath this frontline healthcare gap, there exists another gap: a lack of evidence from consistent research on disability support services and outcomes in rural Australia (Moran et al., 2024). This chapter aims to explore these apparent inequities in rural disability research and outcomes, drawing on four aspects of my own lived experiences, both personally and professionally.

I present myself as a person born with the neurological disease CMT (National Institute of Neurological Disorders and Stroke, 2024) with the early onset variant Type 3 Dejerine-Sottas (Hobbelink et al., 2018). Characterised by its progressive and complex nature, CMT is often associated with limitations in core body functions and reduced mobility (Ferraro et al., 2024). This chapter offers a reflective account of lived experience as a person with disability in rural Australia, alongside the perspective of serving as an elected local government Councillor in rural New South Wales (NSW), directly engaged in the frontline implementation of disability policy (NSW Electoral Commission, 2017). Mine is an unusual narrative, as it is also one that includes lived experience as a researcher into the very disease that I myself have as well as an amplification of the many voices of people with CMT that I encountered across Australia as part of the research project.

The aim of this chapter is to consider observations that were made through these four lenses from 2012 to 2022 – a decade of my life. Emphasis is placed on the importance of identifying the relationship between disability research in rural Australia and the resulting increase in community awareness of chronic, long-term health conditions. This connection highlights the broader impact of research in shaping understanding and responses within rural settings. Rural health research is expected to contribute to addressing existing inequities in disability research and support between rural and metropolitan Australia, while also generating evidence to inform more effective and targeted structural policy responses.

Part 1: Research project on CMT

The transition from lived experience of CMT, beginning in early childhood, to formally investigating the condition through research in 2012, marked a significant shift from personal understanding to scholarly inquiry. In my capacity as Postdoctoral Research Associate at the University of Sydney, funding was secured through a grant awarded by the Australian Government Department of Health to support research in this field. The grant's directive focused on improving the government's understanding of the disease as well as streamlining healthcare delivery. The research project ('the Project') was titled 'Reducing the Burden of Charcot-Marie-Tooth in Australia 2015' (Burns et al., 2016).

This research corresponds to an adjunct project developed by The University of Sydney for the Charcot-Marie-Tooth Association of Australia (CMTAA) under the Chronic Disease Prevention and Service Improvement Fund ('the Fund') (Australian Government Department of Health, 2016). An Australian Government initiative, the programme was administered by the Department of Health and Ageing (Australian Government Department of Health, 2017), which is responsible for community-based services and preventative health measures. In contrast, acute healthcare primarily falls under the jurisdiction of state and territory governments as well as retaining the principal constitutional responsibility for the delivery of health services (General Practice Supervision Australia, 2016).

Programme description and objectives

The Fund was established to support activities designed to address the growing responsibility of chronic disease. Its main objective was to promote targeted actions aimed at chronic disease prevention and service improvements, particularly within the primary care and community sectors. The primary goals were to reduce the rates of preventable mortality and morbidity and maximise the quality of life and overall well-being for individuals affected by chronic disease, from diagnosis through to end-of-life care. Additionally, the Fund sought to alleviate the burden on healthcare and aged care systems and promote evidence-based best practices for the prevention, early detection, treatment and management of chronic diseases (Australian Government Department of Health, 2016). To achieve these objectives and implement the Fund's key principles into practice, it identified the following three priority areas: prevention across the continuum of care, early detection and effective treatment. This approach was designed to ensure integration and continuity of prevention and care in conjunction with individual self-management of both illness and ageing. The main objectives of the Project were derived from the overarching goals of the Fund. It also sought to determine the financial cost of CMT to the government and recommend policies and strategies to better utilise resources within the identified areas of the public sector (Burns et al., 2016).

What is Charcot-Marie-Tooth? Epidemiology

CMT disease is a genetically and clinically diverse group of inherited disorders that affect the peripheral nervous system (Dubourg et al., 2012). It was first described in 1886 by pioneering neurologists Jean-Martin Charcot, Pierre Marie and Howard Henry Tooth (Banchs, 2009). CMT and related disorders represent the most common hereditary neuromuscular conditions globally.

Prevalence estimates fall between 1 in 2,500 and 1 in 1,214 individuals, influenced by factors such as ethnic background and methodological variations in data collection (Saporta, 2014). These estimates correspond to approximately 10,169 individuals in Australia, as per the 2021 Australian Bureau of Statistics Population Census (Australian Bureau of Statistics, 2021b). However, as the landscape of genetics evolves, the algorithms for testing are also likely to change (Tousignant et al., 2014). A hereditary condition, (notwithstanding sporadic cases), CMT can often be identified within extended family groups. Symptoms, severity and age of onset can vary considerably, even among members of the same family and indeed within the same CMT type (Ma et al., 2023).

CMT disrupts the functionality of both motor and sensory nerve pathways (National Institute of Neurological Disorders and Stroke, 2024), specifically the peripheral nerves, which are responsible for transmitting signals from the spinal cord to the extremities. CMT also exhibits a length-dependent pattern of affliction, initially targeting the most distal nerves before progressively affecting more proximal ones. Typical symptoms include progressive muscular weakness in the extremities, structural abnormalities of the hands and feet, reduced or absent tendon reflexes, sensory impairment which may range from mild to severe and chronic neuropathic pain (Krajewski et al., 2000; Peretti et al., 2022). Mobility-related symptoms include foot drop, difficulty in foot elevation, balance problems, a high-stepped gait characterised by frequent tripping or falling and scoliosis (National Institute of Neurological Disorders and Stroke, 2024). Depending on the severity of the disease, symptoms can range from subclinical and/or barely noticeable to significant disability necessitating the use of mobility aids (Nam & Choi, 2019).

Research project initial roll-out

The first major observation made at the time of this study was that 'people with CMT are a motivated group willing to assist researchers and have their voices heard'(Burns et al., 2016). This heightened willingness among people with CMT to share their experiences greatly enhanced the quality of the research data. Additionally, there was considerable interest in the Project from people with CMT living in rural Australia, who demonstrated a notably higher level of enthusiasm for the Project compared to their urban counterparts, which in itself was high.

The Project commenced with primary data through a self-reporting survey, followed by focus group discussions. The criteria stipulated that participants must be over 18 years of age, reside in Australia and possess a formal diagnosis of CMT disease. Family members, caregivers and partners of people with CMT were also invited to engage in the focus groups, which were held at a later date. The survey, titled 'A Survey of Costs, Utility Wellbeing and Management' (hereafter referred to as 'the Survey'), represented the largest known survey conducted for people with CMT in Australia at that time. A primary recruitment of 716 generated 418 usable responses, with 260 returned by hardcopy and 158 completed online. Participants ranged in age from 18 to 96 and included people from all Australian states and territories. Data analysis from the survey identified areas of interest that were used in the second stage of the project to formulate the focus group questions (Burns et al., 2016).

While collating the survey data, it became apparent to the research team that a loose network was forming as news of the research began to spread. Inquiries for additional surveys were requested from individuals beyond the original recruitment database, indicating broader engagement. A considerable number of these requests came from residents living in rural and regional Australia, located in towns and areas unfamiliar to me. This cohort of people also demonstrated a keen interest in participating in the focus groups, an unexpected response that steered the Project in an unforeseen direction. The involvement of rural Australians in both focus groups and surveys offered valuable insights into the distinct challenges of managing neurological conditions in rural contexts (an issue explored in greater detail later in this chapter).

Focus groups

The second phase of data collection involved qualitative focus group interviews conducted at the state branch offices of the CMTAA (Burns et al., 2016). Initially, it was my intention to travel to each state and territory by plane, assuming that I would only need to visit the capital cities. However, due to this unexpected influx of requests from respondents located outside the main metropolitan areas, I felt it was necessary to expand the focus group plan to include regional areas.

Subsequently, the reach of the research was expanded through additional focus groups that were organised and conducted in regional areas beyond the capital cities in each state. These locations included Dalby and Toowoomba in Queensland, Bathurst and Lithgow in NSW, Mildura and Warrnambool in Victoria and

Murray Bridge in South Australia. This new direction for the Project necessitated a major extension of the focus group duration, travel itinerary and budget, as there was now a requirement to visit the many rural inland towns and shires by car to conduct the extra unscheduled focus groups. The focus group format was also modified to include questions pertinent to people with CMT living in rural Australia. Ultimately, this led to an improvement in the study's outcomes, allowing for a larger sample and emphasising the need for research in this underserved area. Rural populations are frequently under-represented in health research due to the additional logistical and financial challenges involved, emphasising the critical need for comprehensive studies that address this persistent knowledge gap (Rolf et al., 2021). In total, this study consisted of twenty-one focus groups held across all states of Australia and the ACT: eight in state/territory capitals and thirteen in rural and regional areas (Burns et al., 2016).

Focus groups were conducted with a total of 178 participants, comprising individuals diagnosed with CMT and their family members (Burns et al., 2016). My lived experience with CMT proved valuable in guiding discussions in contextually appropriate and constructive directions. This experiential knowledge enabled a stronger rapport with participants, thereby enhancing the depth and quality of engagement throughout the research process. Open-ended questions were used to elicit participant responses, fostering a dynamic and responsive discussion environment conducive to in-depth exploration of experiences and perspectives. The comments and narratives provided by participants were subsequently categorised into themes that identified and described the life experiences and daily challenges associated with living with CMT. Such challenges included pain management, lack of access to healthcare professionals, medications, assistive technologies and decisions regarding genetic testing and diagnosis avoidance (Burns et al., 2016).

Focus group data obtained in rural settings made it possible to identify the distinct characteristics of rural lived experience, particularly in relation to the influence of the social determinants of health (Australian Government Australian Institute of Health and Welfare, 2024b). Additionally, rural responses underscored the constraints posed by geographical distance from vital services and the support systems necessary for managing one's disability (Stehlik, 2017). The feedback from the focus group responses presented a broader range of explanatory categories compared to the original survey, with certain rural-specific categories identified. Qualitative and quantitative data from the focus groups and surveys were integrated within a unified research design, through which rural life emerged as a distinct analytical classification.

Genetic testing disparities by remoteness index

Genetic testing and diagnosis are important in identifying an individual's specific CMT subtype to differentiate it from other neuropathies, owing to the potential overlap in symptoms with other neuromuscular disorders. An accurate diagnosis facilitates informed planning for disease progression and potential complications, supports the development of tailored treatment and rehabilitation strategies and allows individuals to prepare for lifestyle modifications that may be necessary in the future. The data can also indicate whether a patient is typical or considered 'unusual for a particular genotype' (Saporta et al., 2011). Individuals diagnosed with CMT may choose to share this information with extended family members, which can raise awareness as well as generate a range of positive outcomes, including earlier detection and intervention (Saporta et al., 2011).

The research results were organised to illustrate the frequency of genetic diagnoses across different national and state locations. A major observation identified was that experiences of CMT differed depending on remoteness, as indicated, among other things, by genetic testing data. This finding was particularly significant, given the relatively high prevalence of CMT. Statistical analysis also identified a direct correlation between lower rates of genetic diagnosis and reduced awareness of CMT in rural communities.

Focus group findings indicated that disparities in CMT diagnosis and awareness could be attributed to a range of contributing factors. Among these factors were the geographical challenges associated with distance (Dorrigan, 2023), a lack of specialist care in rural areas, the necessity to travel to metropolitan areas for affordable access to specialist services and the healthcare professionals' levels of knowledge, commitment, and funding as well as the prevailing attitudes of stoicism and self-sufficiency often found in rural communities (O'Sullivan et al., 2014). These challenges also had much to do with rural residents with CMT exhibiting hesitance to address health concerns in general (Australian Government Department of Health, 2016). Another common theme identified in the focus group discussions was the need for improved communication between newly diagnosed people with CMT and their treating healthcare professionals (Burns et al., 2016). Ultimately, I observed that a positive relationship existed between awareness of the CMTAA and its functions and the likelihood of people seeking formal genetic diagnosis. The following state and territory data derived from the outcomes support this hypothesis (Burns et al., 2016).

The Australian Capital Territory (ACT) had the highest percentage (82%) of genetically tested people with CMT across all Australian states and territories. Moreover, the ACT was the only state/territory where all respondents were able to communicate if they had, or had not, been tested. It is worth mentioning that the ACT does not have a divide between metropolitan and rural areas (Burns et al., 2016).

In NSW, 73% of people with CMT had undergone genetic testing, the second-highest rate in Australia, while 8% of respondents expressed uncertainty regarding their testing status. Survey participants were recruited from the NSW 'inner regional' cities of Orange, Cowra, Bathurst and Lismore, the 'outer regional' city of Parkes and the 'remote area' city of Dubbo. The locations of 148 survey participants were mapped using the Australian Statistical Geography Standard (ASGS) Remoteness Index (Australian Bureau of Statistics, 2023). Analysis of the survey data consistently found that the frequency of CMT diagnoses decreased in line with the ASGS index across all the NSW localities. In the 'major city' of Sydney, 82% of people with CMT were genetically tested, with 12% unsure and 6% untested. Other major urban areas in NSW under the ASGS classification system included Wollongong (covering the entire Illawarra region, Kiama and Shellharbour) and the major Hunter region cities of Newcastle, Lake Macquarie and Maitland. The overall findings of the survey results revealed a higher incidence of uncertainty regarding genetic testing status among individuals with CMT residing in the major cities of NSW compared to those who reported that they had not been tested (Burns et al., 2016).

Access to genetic testing in Queensland was reported to be limited to Brisbane, the state's principal metropolitan centre. Focus groups conducted in regional locations within the state of Queensland (Sunshine Coast and Dalby) revealed that very few neurological specialists in these areas recommended that their patients undertake genetic testing (Burns et al., 2016).

South Australia's genetic testing rates were among the lowest of any Australian state/territory, with only 53% of respondents having undergone testing. However, at the time of this study, the CMTAA was in the process of establishing a well-organised branch in South Australia, and with the addition of this peak advocacy cell, it is likely that testing rates will increase due to recent awareness campaigns promoted through this branch (Burns et al., 2016).

Tasmania reported the lowest genetic testing rate in Australia at 37%, with several individuals indicating that they had travelled to Melbourne to access testing services. This finding highlights a complex range of barriers beyond geographic remoteness, including limited research infrastructure and service availability. Tasmanian focus group participants identified that long delays and poor communication with healthcare professionals were commonplace when compared to their experiences in Sydney and Melbourne, as revealed by the following quote (Burns et al., 2016).

> My GP thought I might have CMT and referred me to a neurologist in Hobart. It was 5 months later and $200 to see the neurologist for 10 minutes. There was no mention of genetic testing.
> Burns et al., 2016, p. 28

On a positive note, the Tasmanian branch of the CMTAA proactively supported individuals newly diagnosed with CMT and facilitated the dissemination of current information on diagnostic procedures and disease management strategies (Burns et al., 2016).

The genetic testing rate for CMT in Victoria was identified as 57%, considerably lower than the rate observed in NSW. As part of the study, a Melbourne-based general practitioner (GP), whose patient cohort included several individuals from the Vietnamese community with CMT, contacted the research team after hearing about the Project. A focus group was held at the GP's clinic. Participants, diagnosed with CMT by different neurologists across Melbourne, arrived with printed copies of their diagnostic letters, seeking further clarification and understanding of their condition (Burns et al., 2016).

A key challenge identified in this focus group was the language barrier, which hindered participants' ability to understand their diagnosis. Test results were provided in English, making it difficult for individuals with limited English proficiency to interpret. As a result, participants expressed uncertainty and confusion regarding the nature of their diagnosis, the implications of their specific CMT subtype and what health outcomes to expect. Some were unsure if CMT was a terminal condition, highlighting a broader lack of accessible post-diagnostic information and support.

The session revealed a systemic gap in care: while specialists in Victoria were diagnosing CMT and identifying specific subtypes, there was an absence of a structured care pathway to support individuals after diagnosis.

An important insight from this experience was the pressing need for neurologists and healthcare providers to collaborate more closely with member-based support organisations. Developing structured post-diagnosis support networks would help address gaps in patient understanding, offer essential resources and enhance the long-term management of CMT. The CMTAA functions as an important network through which individuals with CMT, their families and caregivers can share lived experiences and access peer-informed resources.

In Western Australia, 72% of people with CMT had undergone genetic testing and were generally well informed about their genetic type. Notably, none of the survey participants were uncertain about whether they had been tested. When reviewing the focus group data, I noted that Western Australians were generally well informed about their own genetic testing options and demonstrated a willingness to undergo testing. Additionally, the CMTAA Western Australian state branch organisers maintained a strong and collaborative relationship with neurologists, who actively participated in the Perth capital city branch CMTAA meetings (Burns et al., 2016).

Observations drawn from visiting multiple states and conducting in-person focus groups provided valuable insights into the diverse needs of Australians living with CMT. Notably, 43.2% of individuals with CMT in Australia were unaware of their specific subtype, a significant gap in diagnostic clarity. This state-by-state comparison revealed the unequal access to genetic testing for CMT across Australia, illustrating that geographical location, access to specialists and language proficiency can significantly influence diagnosis. These findings revealed the persistent disparities in healthcare access and emphasised a need for greater awareness, communication and support across both metropolitan and rural areas. Given that genetic testing forms the basis for specialist intervention, such disparities continue to present substantial challenges to the effective diagnosis, treatment and research of CMT in Australia.

Diagnosis aversion

A notable theme that emerged from focus group discussions, including those held in rural locations, was a growing concern among participants about the potential negative consequences of receiving a formal diagnosis. This is a phenomenon referred to as 'diagnosis aversion' (Miller, 2007). A number of participants expressed apprehension that receiving a formal diagnosis would necessitate disclosure to insurance providers, employers and other organisations. Fears of insurance discrimination, bureaucratic hurdles, travel restrictions and threats to job security was an underlying worry. The thinking was that not having a formal diagnosis would allow individuals a degree of plausible deniability. Participants also raised privacy fears related to the protection of genetic information.

Genetic discrimination has emerged in recent years, particularly within the life insurance sector, where the onset of genetic conditions can impact access to and coverage of income-related policies (Adjin-Tettey, 2013). In a conversation outside the focus group, participants shared that they had declined genetic testing due to concerns that their children might face future discrimination, expressing a lack of confidence in the Australian Government's ability to ensure genetic privacy and protection. Apprehensions about insurance policy denial or the arbitrary application of exclusions were compounded by the limited scope of recognised genetic conditions (Adjin-Tettey, 2013). Consequently, the decision to undergo genetic testing has increasingly been framed as an economic consideration (Burns et al., 2016).

Part 2: Management of chronic disease and disability in rural Australia

The 'bush telegraph' and its role in research

The CMTAA, Australia's peak advocacy and information organisation for people with CMT, supported the Project by providing access to a national database of individuals who had expressed willingness to participate in the study (Charcot-Marie-Tooth Association Australia); however, as the Project progressed, it became evident that undertaking research in rural settings also served to increase community awareness. In addition to the unexpectedly high number of survey requests received from individuals in rural Australia, the manner in which these participants became aware of the Project proved particularly revealing. The individuals who made contact were not included in any of the databases provided and would likely not have been identified if they had not independently reached out after learning about the Project through informal channels. Moreover, the response was surprisingly swift. Clusters of survey requests emerged across broad geographic regions, resembling the function of the 'bush telegraph' (Strongman, 2014), an informal communication network characteristic of Australian rural communities through which information spreads rapidly via word of mouth.

It is my view that this 'bush telegraph' phenomenon played an important role in enhancing the research process. The bush telegraph resulted in a heightened willingness among individuals residing in rural areas to engage in the Project in contrast to their metropolitan counterparts. It was not until I became part of that rural community network two years following the conclusion of the Project in 2017 that I fully appreciated how the concept of the bush telegraph operated in practice. This experience contributed to a more nuanced understanding of its role within the context of disability research. The message was clear: rural Australians expressed a strong interest in the continuation of research on CMT to be conducted in their communities (Burns et al., 2016). The operation of the bush telegraph also formed the basis of the first of two case studies to be introduced.

Case study 1: Rural CMT farming family

The first lived experience case study centres on a family residing in regional Victoria who adopted an unconventional approach to managing CMT. Select elements of this case study were incorporated into the Project's final report. Information disseminated through the 'bush telegraph' brought the research team's attention to a large family residing in rural Victoria affected by CMT. Subsequent email correspondence resulted in contact from a family member who expressed interest in participating in the study. It was mutually agreed that a focus group would be conducted on the family's farm. To optimise research outcomes, the focus group was limited solely to members of this extended family and comprised a manageable cohort of fourteen participants.

Participation in focus groups became more approachable over time, as the shared experience of CMT among attendees created an environment that was conducive to open and honest discussions about the challenges and realities of living with the condition. This sense of familiarity was particularly evident upon arrival at the family's farm, where I was welcomed into a kitchen-dining area and joined by several family members. Many visibly exhibited physical signs consistent with CMT. Common clinical features of CMT observed included foot drop, foot deformities such as hammertoes or curled toes, pes cavus (high-arched feet), distal muscle wasting in the lower legs resulting in an 'inverted champagne bottle' appearance, hand atrophy and scoliosis (Adjin-Tettey, 2013). During our conversation, the farm manager gestured toward a AUD 60,000 diesel fuel invoice that happened to be on the table, noting that it represented only a single month of operational costs. This gesture accentuated the scale and complexity of the farming enterprise.

The focus group discussion revealed that until recently, the family had not sought a medical diagnosis, information or treatment for their condition. In fact, no family member had previously heard of CMT. It was only through the 'bush telegraph' that the family became aware of CMT, and subsequently the Project.

Notably, they were unaware that their condition was part of a globally recognised disorder affecting approximately 1 in 2,500 people (Saporta, 2014). Family members had believed it to be a rare, hereditary condition confined to their lineage alone (Burns et al., 2016). Meeting an individual outside their family who both lived with CMT and was conducting research on the condition prompted a highly engaged response. A wide range of questions were raised concerning available support services, projected life expectancy and broader aspects of disease management.

In the absence of formal diagnoses and engagement with allied health services or other support resources, the family adopted a self-directed approach to managing CMT. Nearly all aspects of care were addressed independently, without professional healthcare intervention. Over time, they implemented a range of adaptations within their agricultural practices to accommodate the functional limitations associated with the condition. A notable adaptation was the family's initiative to handcraft custom footwear using their own skills, specifically designed to address clinical manifestations such as pes cavus, hammertoes and other related foot deformities experienced by several family members.

During a tour of the farm, I was shown agricultural equipment valued in the hundreds of thousands of dollars, offering insight into the farm's substantial diesel consumption mentioned earlier. One particularly remarkable example of adaptation involved a tractor that had been manually modified: the accelerator and brake pedals were removed and reversed to accommodate a farmer with CMT, whose left leg retained more strength than his right, thereby enhancing control over the vehicle. When asked whether any professional support had been engaged for this alteration, the family stated that their only 'professional assistance' consisted of a grinder and a welding machine.

At first glance, this case appeared to reflect a rejection of the medical model of disability (Heery & Noon, 2008), with the family opting for self-reliance in managing their own condition. However, it soon became apparent that they had inadvertently fallen through systemic gaps in healthcare provision, and they were not alone. During travel across rural Australia, additional, albeit on a smaller scale, instances of similar isolation were identified. My observations pointed to a significant gap in awareness of CMT, particularly in rural contexts, which required attention. Typically, the responsibility for raising awareness and delivering education about CMT would rest with neurologists, general practitioners, allied health professionals or the CMTAA.

The evolving recognition of CMT in Australia

Engagement with participants through the CMT survey and focus groups, and the sharing of aspects of lived experience, provided valuable insights into the diverse journeys of individuals with CMT and their support networks. Travelling throughout regional and rural Australia deepened my understanding of life beyond the capital cities for people with disability. It was only several years after these visits to rural homes and communities that I began to reflect on the potential role that local government processes could play in addressing persistent gaps in disability awareness across rural Australia.

The lack of awareness of CMT disease among healthcare professionals has remained a persistent theme throughout my life.

Throughout my early childhood in the 1970s and into my formative years extending into the 1980s, it was common for general practitioners and treating physicians at hospitals whom I encountered to possess minimal to no knowledge or understanding of CMT. Further still, interactions with allied health professionals who possessed any familiarity with the condition were even more uncommon. During this time, I received a series of misdiagnoses, including muscular dystrophy, Friedreich's ataxia and even lead poisoning. By the end of the 1980s, a formal diagnosis had yet to be confirmed, although one neurologist expressed a strong suspicion that a variant of CMT might be present.

During the 1990s and early 2000s, I found that limited familiarity with CMT disease remained evident among many general practitioners and resident doctors. Nevertheless, I could see that there was a notable improvement in awareness of the condition across the medical community, particularly among allied health professionals. In 1994, Professor Garth Nicholson, a neurologist recognised for his expertise and leadership in CMT research (Mellor & Miller, 2008), conducted a nerve conduction study and subsequently provided me with a formal diagnosis of a specific CMT subtype (Charcot-Marie-Tooth Association Australia, 2025; Shy et al., 2005). This diagnosis was facilitated through genetic panel testing, a process that, at the time, was becoming increasingly accessible and affordable for both clinicians and patients (McClain, 2021).

Professor Nicholson became a central figure in my medical journey over the decades, often providing critical guidance when other practitioners lacked expertise in CMT. His enduring support played a key role in shaping my care and deepening my understanding of the condition. I remain deeply appreciative of his contributions to CMT research and advocacy, particularly his establishment of the CMTAA in the early 1980s, which has since provided vital support and information to many individuals and families, including my own. As of 2025, based on my lived experience, it is encouraging to see that most allied health professionals now demonstrate at a minimum a basic familiarity with, and for some, a deeper understanding of CMT in clinical practice.

Case study 2: a rural baker's narrative

The second case study features a focus group participant residing in rural Australia, whose occupation was baker and cake decorator. This participant brought a photo album to the focus group containing images of their decorative cakes. Unfortunately, their professional career had been interrupted due to the progression of pes cavus and hammertoes, which had worsened to the point where they were unable to wear footwear necessary to comply with occupational health and safety guidelines.

During the focus group, fellow participants as well as myself were able to relay to the person that foot surgery may be an option. Subsequently, the participant was put in contact with a metropolitan specialist who offered surgical treatment options, allowing the participant to resume their professional baking career. This case, among others, illustrated how the Project was not only raising awareness but also delivered tangible improvements to the lives of people with CMT. It became evident that focus groups functioned as more than just forums for discussion, they also served as vehicles for meaningful change.

Building awareness as a solution to bridging gaps in disability research

As previously noted, disparities in disability support between urban and rural areas remained evident, often reflecting broader inequities in health outcomes. During my time as a researcher engaging with people with disability in rural communities, it became increasingly clear that a key barrier to improved health outcomes was the widespread lack of awareness, not only within the medical profession but across the broader community. This gap in awareness appeared to be deeply intertwined with the social determinants of health, including income, education, nutrition, housing and geographic isolation (Green et al., 2022).

The disadvantages arising from the complex interplay of the social determinants of health are clearly compounded for individuals with CMT residing in rural Australia. Disability intersects with all of these determinants, intensifying existing barriers associated with the management of disability and exacerbating the obstacles in navigating everyday life (Charcot-Marie-Tooth Association Australia, 2025). Contributing factors such as geographic isolation and limited access to specialist diagnostic, treatment and management services contribute further to these barriers. One of the Project's key findings indicated a marked decline in the rate of genetic testing for CMT with increasing geographical remoteness across Australia (Burns et al., 2016).

Drawing from my perspective as both a researcher and a person with CMT, I could see that addressing these disparities required a multifaceted approach centred on awareness, accessibility and tailored support for individuals with CMT in rural Australia. Key strategies include improving education and awareness among healthcare professionals, increasing access to genetic testing and specialist services and developing community-based initiatives to bridge the urban-rural divide in disability support. Additionally, policy interventions that address the broader social determinants of health, in particular economic security, housing and transport, are essential in mitigating the compounded disadvantages faced by individuals with CMT living in rural areas. A final obstacle to consider is the prevailing attitude of stoicism prevalent in many rural communities, resulting in accepting and adapting to disability rather than actively exploring diagnosis, treatment options and available support (Bullock et al., 2010). Addressing these systemic and attitudinal barriers is essential to improving health outcomes and quality of life for people with CMT residing in rural areas.

Future research considerations

The focus groups offered clarity to the survey findings, enabling the interpretation of ambiguous or unexpected quantitative data by exploring participants' underlying reasoning, lived experiences and motivations behind their responses. The groups added contextual richness to the survey's open-ended responses, supporting the identification of new or emerging themes and informing future research directions. In particular, participant feedback underscored the need for practical innovations in assistive technology to enhance the everyday management of CMT as a somewhat complex and little-known disability in a rural Australian setting (Burns et al., 2016).

The project identified a clear research gap in understanding the day-to-day realities of life for rural Australians with CMT. Drawing on my own lived experience while conducting the research, it is my view that future investigations should prioritise two key areas. First, there is a need to increase awareness of CMT and its symptoms within rural communities. Second, research should investigate the development of tailored management strategies specific to rural contexts. One such example is mobility equipment suited for harsh rural environments. A structured support system, together with a well-organised framework, would ideally offer consistent, accessible and effective guidance and assistance for individuals with CMT living in rural areas.

The peak national body, the CMTAA, is well positioned to lead the development of this structured support system, provided it receives adequate and ongoing funding. It has demonstrated a willingness to extend its reach beyond traditional Sydney-based activities, notably through the relocation of its annual seminar to Adelaide, where researchers present to members. As a volunteer-run organisation with limited resources, the CMTAA is governed by a committee of nine individuals, all of whom have personal experience with CMT, either directly or through a family member. The CMTAA is likely to play a central role in advancing future CMT research in Australia and has produced literature emphasising the importance of investigating the experiences of people living with CMT in rural areas (Charcot-Marie-Tooth Association Australia, 2025).

An often overlooked consideration when contemplating future research directions for people with disability in rural Australia is the demographic composition of these regions. Regional areas have a higher proportion of older adults (over 65 years) compared to metropolitan centres (Australian Government Australian

Institute of Health and Welfare, 2024b). Additionally, remote and very remote areas have disproportionately higher Indigenous populations (Australian Government Australian Institute of Health and Welfare, 2024a). Both older Australians and Aboriginal and Torres Strait Islander people experience increased rates of disability. These intersecting demographic factors, combined with the geographic harshness and infrastructure limitations typical of rural and remote communities, complicate the effective management of disability and CMT.

Part 3: Government policy on disability

Tree-change

The unexpected expansion of the Project beyond metropolitan areas marked a pivotal moment in my understanding of rural Australian life. What initially began as a research initiative gradually evolved into a personal journey, eventually leading to a major lifestyle change. In 2016, I relocated from Sydney to Blayney, a small town in the Central West region of NSW. With a population of approximately 3,000 residents (about 8,000 across the broader local government area [LGA]) (Australian Bureau of Statistics, 2021a), Blayney presented a sharp contrast to urban life, characterised by its rural landscapes, close-knit community and strong sense of belonging.

Motivated to integrate quickly into my new surroundings, I actively pursued opportunities to contribute to local life. In 2017, I took a decisive step by running for local government and was subsequently elected as a Councillor for the Blayney Shire Council. This role marked the beginning of a transformative period during which I served for 4.5 years (NSW Electoral Commission, 2017). My tenure coincided with the unprecedented challenges of the COVID-19 pandemic, a time that tested the resilience and adaptability of rural communities and reinforced the essential role of local governance in crisis response.

Beyond my role on council, I also became involved in a range of community initiatives. I served as vice president of Lee Hostel, a local aged care facility, where I gained valuable firsthand insight into the distinct needs of elderly residents in rural Australia (Lee Aged Care Blayney, 2025). Additionally, I chaired the Blayney Shire Council Local Access Advisory Committee (BSC LAAC), later reformed as the Disability Inclusion Working Group (Blayney Shire Council, 2025b). I collaborated with community members, fellow councillors and council staff to implement inclusive policies and support structures. These experiences complemented and deepened the insights that I had previously acquired through my CMT research. Together, these roles provided a practical perspective on pressing disability policy challenges, including a need to improve the accessibility of social and health services in a rural context.

Ultimately, my understanding of rural communities transformed from observation to lived experience. The challenges were tangible and immediate, but so too were the opportunities to effect change, address gaps in disability support and contribute meaningfully to the evolving landscape of rural governance.

The relationship between policy and legislative instruments in New South Wales

The National Disability Strategy (NDS) (Australian Government Department of Social Services, 2024) outlines the Australian

Government's commitment to fulfilling its obligations under the UNCRPD, to which Australia is a signatory (United Nations, 2006). NSW's response to the NDS was the enactment of the Disability Inclusion Act 2014 (DIA 2014) (NSW Government, 2021) as a state-based framework to support the objectives of the NDS. The implementation of these three instruments – the UNCRPD, the NDS and the DIA 2014 – serves as the foundation for the NSW Disability Inclusion Plan (DIP) (NSW Government, 2025).

A key mandate of the NSW DIA 2014 was that communities be inclusive and accessible for people with disabilities. Consequently, under the NSW DIP, all NSW public authorities, including Local Government Councils, are required to have a Disability Inclusion Action Plan (DIAP) in place, ensuring that councils actively promote equal participation for people with disabilities within their communities (NSW Government, 2025). During my tenure as an elected Councillor and chair of the Local Access Advisory Committee, I observed effective disability policy implementation through Blayney Shire Council's DIAP (Blayney Shire Council, 2025).

Local government's role in disability research

As I gained expertise in my role as a local government Councillor and chair of the Local Access Advisory Committee, I was able to reflect on various aspects of my lived experience as a person with a disability. As a Councillor, I drew on my experience in the LGA while also leveraging my lived experience as a researcher to formulate the hypothesis that local governments can and should better serve as a valuable resource in disability research.

As outlined, all 127 local governments in NSW are required by legislation to implement the NDS through a DIAP. I observed that there was limited collaboration between councils, resulting in inconsistencies in DIAP planning and implementation, and that this is primarily due to the absence of a co-ordinated, statewide data collection framework for disability inclusion. At present, data is gathered on an ad hoc basis, driven by what individual councils consider to be useful. To extrapolate meaningful statistical research data and inform future planning, an efficient, centralised and co-ordinated statewide approach is required. Such a structure would also need to include clear guidance on what data to collect, from whom and how. This approach would allow for the accurate measurement of the progress of the state's role in its implementation of the NDS. Additionally, NSW LGAs could explore how to supplement the statistical picture of disability inclusion performance with other resources, such as the Australian Bureau of Statistics.

A further opportunity for conducting health research in rural Australia lies in leveraging the existing community networks and infrastructure maintained by local councils, such as community centres and village halls. The importance of these facilities is often overlooked, as community centres function as hubs for social connection and necessary communication. These centres also play a key role in the aforementioned 'bush telegraph' process. As accessible, trusted and familiar hubs, rural community centres offer valuable opportunities for researchers to collect data on disability and other health-related issues in a way that is relevant and inclusive.

Local council disability-led policy

Local government policy plays a central role in advancing disability inclusion in rural Australia. NSW Local Council's DIAPs serve as a foundational document and strategic framework guiding councils in prioritising accessibility and inclusion in the design, maintenance and management of public buildings and outdoor spaces.

To strengthen the implementation of DIAPs, councils could benefit from engaging design consultants with expertise in disability access and inclusion. Equally important is the allocation of appropriate funding and dedicated attention from both council staff and elected representatives to ensure meaningful progress in accessibility outcomes. However, a major challenge for the majority of rural councils is limited resources allocated to this function. Many regional local governments operate under financial constraints exacerbated by a "one-size-fits-all" funding model, which fails to account for the diverse and specific needs of individual councils in delivering effective disability support services (Blayney Shire Council, 2025a).

Despite these ongoing challenges, local governments operate within a supportive policy framework that enables the advancement of disability research and inclusion initiatives. This framework aligns with both iterations of the NDS, the original 2010–2020 strategy, and the current strategy, known as Australia's Disability Strategy 2021–2031 (Australian Government Department of Health, Disability and Ageing, 2025a). By leveraging these national frameworks, councils are well-positioned to maximise disability accessibility and inclusion outcomes within their communities.

Better policy on state and federal levels of government

In my role as a local government Councillor (Blayney Shire Council, 2025a) and vice president of the aged care facility Lee

Hostel (Lee Aged Care Blayney, 2025), I frequently encountered disability in a broader community context. However, as Chair of the Local Access Advisory Committee, my responsibilities were primarily focused on ensuring disability inclusion. The combination of these roles afforded me an extremely unique lens to closely observe both the challenges and benefits experienced by people with disability living in rural Australia – in particular, the experiences of people with disability in navigating access to state and federally funded services, such as the NDIS, and the systemic challenges and opportunities for access improvement. The NDIS is an Australian government-funded initiative that delivers support and services to individuals with permanent and significant disabilities, enabling access to essential care, therapies and opportunities for community participation (Australian Government Department of Health, 2025). My observations included reported barriers and limitations in accessing such services, thereby identifying critical areas for policy reform and targeted advocacy.

NDIS participants living in rural Australia encounter additional barriers to plan their utilisation of the Scheme compared to their metropolitan counterparts, largely due to limited access to disability support services (Wakely et al., 2023). Research indicates widespread service shortages, particularly in allied health and home maintenance, which often necessitate considerable travel to access essential care (Mavromaras et al., 2018), resulting in financial and logistical burdens. NDIS participants in rural and remote areas are, on average, '15% more likely to face unmet support needs' (Wakely et al., 2023, p. 2) compared to those in urban regions. Compounding this issue, NDIS planners, who are usually based in metropolitan centres, are frequently reported to lack a nuanced understanding of the unique challenges associated with living with a disability in rural contexts (Australian Federation of Disability Organisations [AFDO, 2024]). This disconnect can result in support plans that do not adequately reflect the needs of rural participants, further contributing to plan underutilisation. These persistent challenges emphasise the need for improved strategic planning and expanded service availability to ensure that the NDIS supports people with disability in rural Australia, as made clear by one participant's concise comment:

> ...there was no NDIS physio at the time, so that was hard... then we moved to [rural town 2]. I didn't have a speech pathologist here. So, I had to Skype to Sydney, so that was difficult. It's very limited with speech pathologists. We just need more speechies.
> Mavromaras et al., 2018, p. 75

As of 2025, the division of responsibilities between Federal and State governments continues to overlap, particularly in the implementation of the Multi-Purpose Service (MPS) healthcare model – a jointly funded initiative. As such, state-funded hospitals and the jointly funded MPS's provide disability diagnosis and treatment, transport to and from rural communities, access to specialised treatments and allied health workers such as occupational therapists and bulk-billing doctors (NSW Government NSW Health, 2025).

Conclusion

This chapter examines disparities in disability support, healthcare access and awareness between rural and metropolitan Australia, with a particular focus on CMT disease. Over a 10-year period,

I observed how geographic isolation, limited access to specialist services and broader social determinants of health intensified the challenges experienced by people with disability living in rural Australia. These inequities were further exacerbated by the lack of co-ordinated research efforts and data collection, which inhibited the development of essential services and the utilisation of resources.

The Project examined the critical role of local government in advancing disability inclusion, particularly through the implementation of DIAPs. It brought to light inconsistent application across councils, which underscored the need for a co-ordinated, statewide strategy to achieve more effective and equitable policy outcomes. Similarly, the NDIS inadequately serviced people with disability living in rural areas, which limited rural participants' ability to make full use of their support plans. Case studies identified significant gaps in awareness, with some families uninformed of their CMT condition and others encountering considerable difficulty accessing supports. Barriers to genetic testing, including fears of discrimination and a lack of post-diagnosis support, further illustrate the challenges experienced by individuals with disabilities in rural settings.

To address the above-mentioned issues, there is a need for individualised management strategies, improved availability of rural disability services, co-ordinated statewide data collection and the development of community-based support networks. Targeted research that draws on lived experience also warrants greater investment. Bridging the identified policy and service gaps will require an ongoing collaborative effort between researchers, people with lived experience of disability, policymakers, healthcare professionals and advocacy organisations such as the CMTAA. In conclusion, a multifaceted, community-driven approach will support the advancement of equitable health outcomes and an inclusive support system for people with disabilities living in rural Australia.

References

Adjin-Tettey, E. (2013). Potential for genetic discrimination in access to insurance: Is there a dark side to increased availability of genetic information? *Alberta law review*, *50*(3), 577–614. https://doi.org/10.29173/alr97

Australian Bureau of Statistics. (2021a). *Blayney: 2021 Census All Persons QuickStats*. Retrieved 1 August from https://abs.gov.au/census/find-census-data/quickstats/2021/LGA10850

Australian Bureau of Statistics. (2021b). *Population: Census. Information on sex and age*. Retrieved 1 August from https://www.abs.gov.au/statistics/people/population/population-census/latest-release

Australian Bureau of Statistics. (2023). *Remoteness Areas - Australian Statistical Geography Standard (ASGS) Edition 3*. Retrieved August 2 from https://www.abs.gov.au/statistics/standards/australian-statistical-geography-standard-asgs-edition-3/jul2021-jun2026/remoteness-structure/remoteness-areas

Australian Federation of Disability Organisations (AFDO). (2024). *NDIS participant experience in Rural, Regional & Remote Australia Submission to the Joint Standing Committee on the National Disability Insurance Scheme* Retrieved August 2 from https://afdo.org.au/wp-content/uploads/2024/03/2024_03-AFDO-Sub-NDIS-RRR-Final-March-2024.pdf

Australian Government Australian Institute of Health and Welfare. (2024a). *Profile of First Nations people*. https://www.aihw.gov.au/reports/australias-welfare/profile-of-indigenous-australians

Australian Government Australian Institute of Health and Welfare. (2024b). *Rural and remote health*. Retrieved August 3 from https://www.aihw.gov.au/reports/rural-remote-australians/rural-and-remote-health

Australian Government Department of Health. (2016). *Public Health and Chronic Disease Grant Program – Guidelines*. Retrieved August 2 from https://www.health.gov.au/sites/default/files/documents/2019/09/public-health-and-chronic-disease-grant-program-guidelines_0.pdf

Australian Government Department of Health. (2017). *Budget 2016–17 Flexible Funds Transition*. Retrieved August 2 from www.aph.gov.au/-/media/Estimates/ca/bud1819/Tabled_Documents/Health/29_May_2018/Department_of_Health_Budget_201617_Flexible_Funds_Transition__tabled_29_May_2018.pdf?la=en&hash=24B94FF81125560C3BB1DCF9CED7E566B1656755

Australian Government Department of Health, Disability and Ageing. (2025). *National Disability Insurance Scheme reforms and reviews*. Retrieved August 3 from https://www.health.gov.au/topics/disability-and-carers/reforms-and-reviews

Australian Government Department of Health, Disability and Ageing. (2025a). Australia's Disability Strategy. Retrieved October 9 from https://www.health.gov.au/our-work/australias-disability-strategy#australias-disability-strategy-20212031

Banchs, I., Casasnovas, C., Alberti, A., De Jorge, L., Povedano, M., Montero, J., Martinez-Matos, J.A. & Volpini, V. . (2009). Diagnosis of Charcot-Marie-Tooth Disease. Journal of Biomedicine and Biotechnology.

Blayney Shire Council. (2025). *Blayney Shire Council*. Retrieved August 3 from https://www.blayney.nsw.gov.au/

Blayney Shire Council. (2025a). *Committees of Council - Local Access Advisory Committee (now known as the Disability Inclusion*

Working Group). Retrieved August 3 from https://www.blayney.nsw.gov.au/council/council-meetings/committees-of-council

Bullock, S., Long, R., & Thompson, L. (2010). *A snapshot of men's health in regional and remote Australia*. Australian Institute of Health and Welfare.

Burns, J., Denton, S., Poynten J., & J., S. (2016). *Reducing the Health Burden of Charcot-Marie-Tooth in Australia 2015*. https://cmtaustralia.org.au/wp-content/uploads/2020/04/reducing-health-burden-of-CMT-Aust.pdf

Charcot-Marie-Tooth Association Australia. (2025). *Diagnosing CMT*. Retrieved August 3 from https://www.cmtausa.org/understanding-cmt/diagnosing-cmt/

Dorrigan, A. (2023). 'The tyranny of distance': rural health inequities persist. *News GP Professional*. https://www1.racgp.org.au/newsgp/professional/the-tyranny-of-distance-rural-health-inequities-pe

Dubourg, O., Brice, A., & LeGuern, E. (2012). Charcot–Marie–Tooth diseases. In N. Wood (Ed.), *Neurogenetics: A Guide for Clinicians* (pp. 166–187). Cambridge University Press. https://doi.org/DOI: 10.1017/CBO9781139087711.012

Ferraro, F., Calafiore, D., Curci, C., Fortunato, F., Carantini, I., Genovese, F., Lucchini, G., Merlo, A., Ammendolia, A., & de Sire, A. (2024). Effects of intensive rehabilitation on functioning in patients with mild and moderate Charcot–Marie-tooth disease: a real-practice retrospective study. *Neurological Sciences*, *45*(1), 289–297. https://link.springer.com/article/10.1007/s10072-023-06998-0

General Practice Supervision Australia. (2016). *FACT SHEET: Organisation of the Australian Health Care System*. Retrieved August 2 from https://gpsa.org.au/factsheet-1-6-organisation-of-the-australian-health-care-system/

Green, H., Fernandez, R., & MacPhail, C. (2022). Well-being and social determinants of health among Australian adults: A national cross-sectional study. *Health & Social Care in the Community, 30*(6), e4345–e4354. https://onlinelibrary.wiley.com/doi/10.1111/hsc.13827

Heery, E., & Noon, M. (2008). *A dictionary of human resource management*. OUP Oxford.

Hobbelink, S. M., Brockley, C. R., Kennedy, R. A., Carroll, K., de Valle, K., Rao, P., Davis, M. R., Laing, N. G., Voermans, N. C., & Ryan, M. M. (2018). Dejerine–Sottas disease in childhood—Genetic and sonographic heterogeneity. *Brain and Behavior, 8*(4), e00919. https://onlinelibrary.wiley.com/doi/10.1002/brb3.919

Krajewski, K. M., Lewis, R. A., Fuerst, D. R., Turansky, C., Hinderer, S. R., Garbern, J., Kamholz, J., & Shy, M. E. (2000). Neurological dysfunction and axonal degeneration in Charcot–Marie–Tooth disease type 1A. *Brain, 123*(7), 1516–1527. https://academic.oup.com/brain/article-abstract/123/7/1516/380271?redirectedFrom=fulltext

Lee Aged Care Blayney. (2025). Roshana Retrieved August 3 from https://www.roshana.com.au/aged-care/lee-aged-care/

Ma, M., Li, Y., Dai, S., Chu, M., Sun, L., Liu, L., & Zhou, J.-C. (2023). A meta-analysis on the prevalence of Charcot–Marie–Tooth disease and related inherited peripheral neuropathies. *Journal of neurology, 270*(5), 2468–2482. https://link.springer.com/article/10.1007/s00415-023-11559-8

Mavromaras, K., Moskos, M., Mahuteau, S., Isherwood, L., Goode, A., Walton, H., Smith, L., Wei, Z., & Flavel, J. (2018). Evaluation of the NDIS.

McClain, T. F. (2021). The Evolution and Practical Application of Genetic Testing. *The Robins Kaplan Justice Report*. https://www.robinskaplan.com/newsroom/insights/the-evolution-and-practical-application-of-genetic-testing

Mellor, L., & Miller, J. (2008). Faculty of medicine online museum and archive. *Australia: The University of Sydney*.

Miller, P. S. (2007). Genetic testing and the future of disability insurance: thinking about discrimination in the genetic age. *The Journal of Law, Medicine & Ethics*, *35*(2_suppl), 47–51. https://journals.sagepub.com/doi/abs/10.1111/j.1748-720X.2007.00152.x

Moran, A., Bulkeley, K., Johnsson, G., Tam, E., & Maloney, C. (2024). Models of governance of disability therapy support workers in rural and remote settings: a systematic scoping review. *International Journal of Environmental Research and Public Health*, *21*(6), 693. https://www.mdpi.com/1660-4601/21/6/693

Nam, S. H., & Choi, B.-O. (2019). Clinical and genetic aspects of Charcot-Marie-Tooth disease subtypes. *Precision and Future Medicine*, *3*(2), 43–68. https://pfmjournal.org/journal/view.php?doi=10.23838/pfm.2018.00163

National Institute of Neurological Disorders and Stroke. (2024). *Charcot-Marie-Tooth disease*. Retrieved August 3 from https://www.ninds.nih.gov/health-information/disorders/charcot-marie-tooth-disease

National Rural Health Alliance. (2023). *Rural Health in Australia Snapshot 2023*. https://www.ruralhealth.org.au/rural-health-in-australia-snapshot/

NSW Electoral Commission. (2017). *Results by local government area: Blayney: Councillor: Summary of Group and Candidate First Preference Votes*. Retrieved August 3 from https://pastvtr.elections.nsw.gov.au/LGE2017/blayney/councillor/summary.htm

NSW Government. (2021). *Disability Inclusion Act 2014 No 41.*. https://legislation.nsw.gov.au/view/whole/html/inforce/current/act-2014-041

NSW Government. (2025). *NSW Disability Inclusion Plan*. https://dcj.nsw.gov.au/community-inclusion/disability-and-inclusion/nsw-disability-inclusion-plan.html

NSW Government NSW Health. (2025). *Hospitals and health services*. Retrieved August 3 from https://www.health.nsw.gov.au/Hospitals/Pages/default.aspx

O'Sullivan, B. G., Joyce, C. M., & McGrail, M. R. (2014). Rural outreach by specialist doctors in Australia: a national cross-sectional study of supply and distribution. *Human resources for health, 12*(1), 50. https://human-resources-health.biomedcentral.com/articles/10.1186/1478-4491-12-50

Peretti, A., Squintani, G., Taioli, F., Tagliapietra, M., Cavallaro, T., & Fabrizi, G. M. (2022). Neuropathic pain in Charcot–Marie-Tooth disease: A clinical and laser-evoked potential study. *European Journal of Pain, 26*(4), 929–936. https://onlinelibrary.wiley.com/doi/10.1002/ejp.1922

Rolf, F., Campbell, N., Thompson, S., & Argus, G. (2021). Australians' experience of the COVID-19 pandemic: Advantages and challenges of scaling up qualitative research using large-scale rapid analysis and building research capacity across rural Australia. *International Journal of Qualitative Methods, 20,* 16094069211051937. https://journals.sagepub.com/doi/10.1177/16094069211051937

Saporta, A. S., Sottile, S. L., Miller, L. J., Feely, S. M., Siskind, C. E., & Shy, M. E. (2011). Charcot-Marie-Tooth disease subtypes and genetic testing strategies. *Annals of neurology, 69*(1), 22–33. https://onlinelibrary.wiley.com/doi/10.1002/ana.22166

Saporta, M. A. (2014). Charcot-Marie-Tooth disease and other inherited neuropathies. *CONTINUUM: Lifelong Learning in Neurology, 20*(5), 1208–1225. https://continuum.aan.com/doi/10.1212/01.CON.0000455885.37169.4c

Shy, M., Blake, J., Krajewski, K., Fuerst, D., Laura, M., Hahn, A., Li, J., Lewis, R., & Reilly, M. (2005). Reliability and validity of the CMT neuropathy score as a measure of disability. *Neurology, 64*(7), 1209–1214. https://www.neurology.org/doi/abs/10.1212/01.WNL.0000156517.00615.A3

Stehlik, D. (2017). Rurality, disability and place identity. In *Disability and Rurality* (pp. 69–80). Routledge. https://www.taylorfrancis.com/chapters/edit/10.4324/9781315577340-6/rurality-disability-place-identity-daniela-stehlik

Strongman, L. (2014). *Bush telegraph: readings in writing.* Cambridge Scholars Publishing.

Tousignant, R., Trepanier, A., Shy, M. E., & Siskind, C. E. (2014). Genetic testing practices for Charcot–Marie–Tooth type 1A disease. *Muscle & nerve*, *49*(4), 478–482. https://onlinelibrary.wiley.com/doi/abs/10.1002/mus.23991

Convention on the Rights of Persons with Disabilities, (2006). https://www.ohchr.org/en/instruments-mechanisms/instruments/convention-rights-persons-disabilities

Wakely, L., Green, E., Little, A., Fisher, K., Wakely, K., Currie, K., & Wolfgang, R. (2023). The lived experience of receiving services as a National Disability Insurance Scheme participant in a rural area: Challenges of choice and control. *Australian Journal of Rural Health*, *31*(4), 648–658. https://onlinelibrary.wiley.com/doi/10.1111/ajr.13000

7 The lived experience of neurodivergence in academic research studies: A neuro-affirming methodology

Jayne Garrod

Introduction

> Nothing about us without us
>
> (Charlton, 1998, in Barnes, 2020)

The experience of childbirth and parenting is transformative for all new parents; however, for some, it can be a time of trepidation and uncertainty. Disabled birth parents often experience additional barriers to those faced by non-disabled parents. Redshaw et al. (2013) note that women with disabilities often experience multiple oppressions and forms of discrimination, restricting their ability to achieve full societal participation. While the literature on parenting neurodivergent children is abundant, the lived experiences of parents identifying as neurodivergent is scarce (Redshaw et al., 2013).

While the topic of neurodivergence is slowly gaining traction in academia, health settings and within the wider public sphere, understandings and reactions vary and are frequently contested (Kapp, 2020). However, in recent years, the landscape has shifted towards understanding neurodivergence in social terms of human rights and identity as opposed to a pathological deficit in need of treatment and cure. Similar to the critical disability and mad studies movements, 'a politics of neurological diversity recognises power inequalities between people differently situated in relation to neurology, comparable with social stratifications such as class, gender, and ethnicity' (Rosqvist et al., 2020). Viewed through a neuroaffirming lens, lived experience is centred and hegemonic views of neurodivergence are countered and resisted.

My PhD thesis entitled 'The lived experiences of neurodivergent birthing people in Australia: A qualitative, reflexive analysis' focuses on the lived childbirth and parenting experiences of birth parents identifying as neurodivergent. It aims to better understand the experience of neurodivergent mothers and families and to amplify the voices of a marginalised and often misunderstood group. In this chapter, I aim to discuss the existing – albeit sparse – research on the lived childbirth and parenting experiences of neurodivergent (Autistic and ADHD) mothers/birthing parents. I then discuss the concepts of insider and participatory research, noting the benefits and challenges of each. I finally discuss ways in which I aim to mediate the challenges of producing insider and participatory research as a PhD researcher and examine the implications for policymaking.

The language of neurodiversity and its uses

The term 'neurodiversity' was coined collaboratively in 1998 by sociologist Judy Singer, journalist Harvey Blume and other members of an autism advocacy email list, and was thereafter incorporated into the lexicon of the fledgling autism advocacy movement (Kapp, 2020; Pellicano & Den Houting, 2022). Its original meaning was simply an acknowledgement of the diversity in human brains, broadly conceptualising such varied conditions as autism, ADHD, Tourette's syndrome, dyslexia and dyscalculia under its umbrella. In some conceptions, it also includes conditions such as schizophrenia, hearing voices, bipolar, Down syndrome and dementia; however, this is contested (Kapp, 2020). The neurodivergence paradigm rejects the biomedical model's notion of neurodivergent conditions as biological impairments and deficits, instead building upon the social model of disability which understands disability as the result of an environment whose structures create barriers for people with impairments (Oliver, cited in Watson & Vehmas, 2020). The term 'neurodivergent' refers to an individual or individuals whose neurodevelopment differs from those considered 'neurotypical', that is, those whose neurodevelopment is considered normative, while the term 'neurodiverse' describes a collective of mixed neurotypical and neurodivergent brains (Pellicano & Den Houting, 2022).

The contemporary neurodivergence paradigm considers the complex intersections and structures that both disadvantage and benefit neurodivergent individuals in a myriad of ways. It advocates for a framework of social inclusion that acknowledges people's differences and agentic capacity as individuals, whilst celebrating the unique and diverse societal contributions of neurodivergent brains (Kapp, 2020).

However, the neurodiversity movement has faced some critique from academics, health professionals and parents of Autistic children for being 'unrepresentative and divisive' (Kapp, 2020, p. vi). Two of the primary arguments made by opponents are that it is not inclusive of people with more significant impairments, whilst some stanchly constructivist social science and humanities academics have suggested the movement is biologically reductionist. A third argument asserts that the terms 'neurotypical' and 'neurodivergent' are divisive and dichotomising, enabling an 'in group' and 'out group' mentality (Russell, 2020, p. 288). A full exploration of the critiques levelled at the neurodiversity movement are outside the scope of this chapter. Suffice to say that my positionality as a neurodivergent researcher aligns with that of the neurodiversity movement, which not only makes compelling arguments about the nature of neurological diversity and its implications for scientific research and understanding, but champions the notion of societal inclusivity eschewing the imperative of the medical model of disability to find a cure for this perceived deviance/deficiency (Kapp, 2020; Pellicano & den Houting, 2022). For those of us who have spent a lifetime feeling strange or deficient, the neurodiversity movement offers the hope of acceptance and equity. daVanport (2019, p. 150) writes:

> Out of Searching Came Community: neurodiversity soon became something that I intimately understood as the all-inclusive acceptance of every neurological difference without exception. I further came to appreciate that neurodiversity didn't leave anyone out. Even the opponents of this concept reaped the benefits of the work by neurodiversity activists. It didn't matter whether they agreed with the concept or not, they personally benefited. Furthermore, their children did as well, as the specific premise of neurodiversity is full and equal inclusion.

The personal is indeed political, and as numerous academics, advocates, and others have noted, it is possible to be cognisant of the disabling societal barriers neuronormative society presents to neurodivergent people, acknowledging the wide diversity in neurodivergent conditions and presentations, while simultaneously being committed to a paradigm shift in terms of societal understandings of neurodivergence. Following other social justice movements, the neurodiversity movement recognises the importance of an intersectional approach which understands that neurodiversity is compounded by other forms of societal oppression such as race/ethnicity, class, gender and sexuality, and works to ameliorate these oppressions (Kapp, 2020; Giwa Onaiwu, 2019). It is therefore imperative to amplify the voices of neurodivergent people, particularly those from further marginalised communities.

The ways in which historical societal conceptions of neurodivergence, and particularly autism, have shifted over the course of the last 100 years have been extensively documented. Steve Silberman's (2016) influential historical analysis of Autism,

Neurotribes, discusses in depth the varying medical and societal paradigms that have dominated Autism psychology, research and practice. In the twentieth century, these ranged from explicitly eugenicist discourses (p. 120) and parental blame (p. 206) to harsh behavioural modification techniques based on psychological methods of operant conditioning (p. 305–310). By the turn of the twenty-first century, a myriad of pseudoscientific alternative treatments were offered as potential 'cures' (365). Common to all these is the prevailing notion of autism as a 'debilitating' and undesirable condition (p. 283) in need of intense management in the hope of overcoming and eliminating Autistic behaviours. The rise of the neurodiversity movement (p. 501–504) has empowered and emancipated Autistic people and their families from bleak and paternalistic conceptions of autism to the idea that Autistic people can live fulfilling, autonomous lives that don't depend on hopes of recovery (p. 504).

However, notions of 'curing' autism persist. Garcia (2021) discusses problematic contemporary societal discourses, including criminally profiling Autistics and spreading misinformation. He notes that three quarters of research funding in America goes towards discovering the 'root causes' of autism and the 'best ways to treat' Autistic people, while only 6% is used for improving services and supports (p. xiv). Donald Trump has been quoted as spreading misinformation and disinformation in terms of the (debunked) connection between vaccination and autism, and furthermore, referring to autism as an 'epidemic' (p. xii). Trump's rhetoric, as stated on Twitter and CNN, extended to his presidential campaign:

> On April 2, 2017, Trump's presidential proclamation for World Autism Day read "My Administration is committed to promoting greater knowledge of [autism spectrum disorders] and encouraging innovation that will lead to new treatments and cures for autism."
>
> Garcia, 2020, p. 239

It is with all this in mind that I commenced my PhD research focusing on the lived experiences of birth parents identifying as neurodivergent. I have undertaken sociological research in the past in the field of childbirth, maternity care and birth trauma, so that is familiar territory. After discovering my own neurodivergence whilst completing a qualifying social work master's degree and working in the field of disability support, I became increasingly interested in the birth and parenting experiences of neurodivergent mothers/birthing people; in fact, I would regularly find myself musing about doing a PhD on the topic. I aim to contribute to the sizable gap in the scholarly literature on the lived experiences of these parents in terms of their *own* experiences of neurodivergence rather than that of parenting their neurodivergent children, of which there is much written. My positionality as a mother who has given birth twice and who identifies as 'AuDHD' (Autistic and ADHD) aligns with the concept of 'insider research', in which the researcher is a part of the community under investigation and possesses a level of knowledge of the community and its members due to lived experience (Greene, 2014; Kirpitchenko & Voloder, 2014). As Pellicano and Den Houting (2022) note, previous research in the United Kingdom reveals that Autistic people and their families have been frequently disappointed in research projects in which they have felt objectified and devoid of agency, often having little to no access to the results of the study in which they participated. It is thus crucial to situate research and policy objectives in contexts that are not only meaningful to neurodivergent people and communities, but which engage neurodivergent people as researchers and coresearchers.

I knew very little about participatory research initially; however, upon doing further reading, I was fascinated and wanted to incorporate this into my thesis. Nevertheless, given the various structural constraints of postgraduate research – and the fact I was already well into my second year and had already changed topic and supervision team once – I decided after discussing the matter with my supervisors to remain with my original (well, *revised*) traditional qualitative research model conducting semi-structured interviews with twelve to fifteen neurodivergent mothers/birth parents recruited mostly from various neurodivergent-focused Facebook groups. That said, my objective is to utilise my insider status reflexively to attempt to negotiate the research process in order to afford participants as much opportunity as possible to amplify their voices and to have meaningful input.

My aims and research questions are:

- To understand the lived experiences of an often-marginalised group, whilst being mindfully aware of differences in identity perception and understandings of what constitutes being 'disabled'.
- To illuminate areas in which neurodivergence is useful or life-enhancing.
- To exert reflexivity regarding the researcher's insider status to assist in amplifying the voices of participants.

- To uncover policy gaps and make salient recommendations for inclusive policymaking.

This latter point is important because it connects research focused on lived experience to policy, reframing the 'problem of autism' (Stace, 2011) in terms of the human rights and support needs of Autistic individuals, as stated by Autistic people themselves.

Note on language and inclusion criteria

Throughout this paper, I utilise the 'identity-first' term 'Autistic' or 'Autistic person' rather than the increasingly outdated 'person-first' term 'person with autism' as preferred by some scholars and clinicians, to reflect the preference of the majority of the Autistic community (Chown, 2017; Kapp, 2020). In line with this, I capitalise the identity-first proper adjective 'Autistic' as it pertains to Autistic individuals as a mark of respect as noted by autism advocacy organisation Amaze (2024). I will, however, use person-first terms when directly citing an author or text. Similarly, I will use 'ADHDer' or 'AuDHDer' when discussing my own experiences; however, as the majority of the published literature used 'person/people with ADHD', I will use that language for purposes of clarity.

Considering the multiple barriers to autism and ADHD diagnosis in Australia (Senate Community Affairs References Committee, 2023; De Broize et al., 2022), I wanted to ensure that participation in my research was as equitable as possible; hence, recruitment criteria states that participants may be professionally or self-diagnosed.

Language used to describe pregnant people/women and mothers/parents will alternate between gendered terms (women, mother) and gender-diverse terms (birthing person, birth parent) to best facilitate inclusion.

Neurodivergent mothers and birthing people

There is extensive interdisciplinary research on childbirth and parenting worldwide. Despite varying opinions on the best methods for childbirth and parenting, it is generally accepted that everyone has the right to a safe birthing environment where they can exercise agency and control. Disabled birth parents often encounter additional obstacles to this objective. The World Health Organization (2022) reports that disabled individuals frequently face stigma and other barriers in the healthcare and maternity care system, including insufficient knowledge or negative attitudes from healthcare providers, discrimination and inaccessible facilities. These issues can lead to feelings of exclusion, otherness and a lack of trust in healthcare providers and systems – factors essential for a positive birthing experience.

The existent literature on people with ADHD is negligible, while that on neurodivergence comprising of two or more (multiple) neurodivergences is non-existent. Scarcely any attention is given to the lived experiences of birth/birthing parents who identify as being both Autistic and ADHD – commonly and colloquially known as 'AuDHDers' (Hinze et al., n.d). This constitutes a monumental gap in the research, which my current research aims to rectify! This is crucially important, considering the rapidly increasing prevalence of diagnosis and/or identification of mixed neurodivergence both in Australia and globally (Sutherland, 2024). It is imperative for policymakers to 'hear' the voices of neurodivergent birthing people, particularly considering recent parliamentary inquiries such as the Select Committee on Birth Trauma (Parliament of NSW, 2023). Various experiences of birth trauma have been apparent in the literature on neurodivergent birthing experiences (Stuart & Reynolds, 2024; Donovan, 2020). The consultation draft of the 'National Autism Roadmap' (Australian Government Department of Health and Aged Care, 2024), despite an extensive consultation and codesign process with Autistic adults, pays scant attention to the needs of Autistic parents other than in their capacity as carers of Autistic children. Due to this lack of mixed identification/dual diagnosis in the literature and policy, this section first considers the sparse literature on mothers/birthing people with ADHD, before moving on to the research on Autistic mothers/birthing people.

Attention-deficit/hyperactivity disorder

Despite having a reported prevalence of 2.5% in adults worldwide (Walsh et al., 2022), research on birthing people with ADHD is scant. What exists is drawn primarily from the disciplines of obstetrics, medicine, nursing or psychology, and commonly framed through a pathological deficit model that focuses attention solely on risks and health complications associated with the condition. Walsh et al. (2022) acknowledge the paucity of research in the perinatal period, arguing that this requires remediating considering ADHD is associated with a variety of comorbidities. This includes 'depression, anxiety and accidents', placing those with the condition at greater risk of negative life outcomes with increased likelihood of mental health issues 'associated with increased pregnancy and birth complications' (Walsh et al., 2022 p. 2). Their study revealed higher rates of every medical condition that was tested for in patients with ADHD, with the authors highlighting the importance of this for informing clinicians treating such patients. Additionally, Walsh et al. (2022 p. 2–3) assert that there is an increased likelihood of women with ADHD, who are taking stimulant medication, experiencing unplanned pregnancies. This issue is explored by Poulton et al. (2018) who note that while ADHD stimulant use and prescribing was low during pregnancy (3.5%), stimulant use was associated with 'small increases in the risk of some adverse pregnancy outcomes' (p. 377). A report by Krewson (2023) cited an increased risk (24%) of mothers with ADHD of developing postpartum depression compared to those without ADHD, while Fuller-Thomson et al. (2016) state that women in general with ADHD were three times more likely to experience conditions, including chronic pain, insomnia, generalised anxiety disorder, suicidal ideation and experience sexual abuse. Additionally, they note that these women are twice as likely to experience 'substance abuse, current smoking, depressive disorders, severe poverty and childhood physical abuse in comparison with women without ADHD' (p. 918). Finally, Samuel et al. (2022, p. 309) observe the potential of recent improvements in autism awareness to similarly inform the needs of women and birthing people with other neurodivergent conditions such as ADHD.

Autistic mothers and birthing people

The Diagnostic and Statistical Manual of Mental Disorders fifth edition (DSM-5)) defines autism as 'Persistent deficits in communication and social interaction across multiple contexts' (American Psychiatric Association, 2013, p. 50). It is considered to be a lifelong neurodevelopmental difference; however, diagnosis requires symptoms to have been present from childhood. In the DSM V, the term 'autism' is used to cover the entirety of pre-DSM V diagnoses, including Asperger syndrome, autism spectrum disorder and pervasive developmental disorder, among others (Chown, 2017). The prevalence of autism is hard to establish due to barriers to diagnosis and changing understandings of the nature and presentation of autism (De Broize et al., 2022); however, Australian Bureau of Statistics data recorded 164,000 Australians with an Autism diagnosis in 2015, an increase of 42.1% since 2012, with the vast majority of those diagnosed being young males (Australian Bureau of Statistics, 2020). However, while there are currently no figures available on the number of Autistic parents in Australia, it is likely that actual numbers are higher. This is possibly due to lack of autism awareness among healthcare providers and financial and other barriers to diagnosis and healthcare faced by Autistic adults in Australia (Arnold et al., 2024; Rasheed, 2023).

Childbirth

Research on Autistic mothers and birthing people is scant, although this is beginning to change. Existent literature reveals a range of strengths and challenges common to Autistic birth parents in terms of both childbirth and parenting experience. Autistic mothers have often been reluctant to disclose their autism to health professionals, citing concerns of negative judgement and stigma (Pohl et al., 2020). A study by Lum et al. (2014) revealed that 75% of participants who revealed their diagnosis had received a negative response, while participants in the research by Hampton et al. (2022) felt professionals were dismissive of their experiences. Hampton et al. identified additional challenges for Autistic mothers in terms of communication and sensory barriers as well as deficits in health professionals' understandings of autism. Sensory sensitivities are common in Autistic adults, with research indicating prevalence at over 90%. Autistic women have reported greater sensory sensitivities than both non-Autistic women and Autistic men (Samuel et al., 2022). Talcer et al. (2023) note that pregnancy heightened the sensory sensitivities of some study participants with such aspects as foetal movement, nausea and heightened visual processing considered distressing.

Sensory experience of light, sound, touch and smell were often heightened in participants in four qualitative studies reporting a significant increase in anxiety throughout childbirth, as discussed in a systematic review by Samuel et al. (2022). Hampton et al. (2022) note that some Autistic participants found the sensory environment of the hospital more stressful than the physiological experience of pain (p. 1168) and found the postnatal maternity ward replete with noise of visitors and crying babies challenging. Some mothers experience sensitivities or aversion to sensations associated with breastfeeding; however, according to Pohl et al. (2020), the majority of Autistic mothers (80%) in their study were able to successfully breastfeed.

Communication issues emerged as another prevailing theme in the literature. Many study participants found communication with professionals difficult due to factors such as lack of autism awareness, perceived negative judgement and communication differences between neurodivergent and neurotypical people. While the medical model argues that Autistic people experience impairments in social communication, the 'double empathy problem' theory arising from a social model perspective argues that neurodivergent and neurotypical people have different communication styles, resulting in difficulty empathising with one another (Mitchell et al., 2021). Autistic women have commonly reported a lack of clear, direct communication from health professionals during pregnancy and childbirth, resulting in misunderstandings, confusion and experience of significant anxiety (Pohl et al., 2020; Hampton et al., 2022).

Several recommendations have been made regarding better ways to support Autistic mothers and birthing people in the perinatal period based on the experiences of these mothers. These include such factors as a need for clear communication, improved continuity of care and vastly improved understanding of the sensory and communication needs of Autistic people. Talcer et al. (2023, p. 846) suggest supporting pregnant Autistic people with occupational therapy to develop 'tailored sensory strategies', further noting that lack of accommodation of Autistic individuals' needs should be viewed as contrary to the Disability Discrimination Act (2010). Hampton et al. (2022) argue for sensory accommodations during childbirth such as dimming of lights, noise reduction, providing a private room where possible and increased awareness among health professionals not only of some of the challenges, but also of the strengths Autistic people possess. This may include in the maternity provision context, increased aptitude for knowledge and research enabling better childbirth preparation and understanding of their own sensory and other needs resulting in the development of coping strategies (Talcer et al., 2023). Better understanding of support needs and improved neurodivergence awareness could significantly reduce the anxiety and overwhelm Autistic women frequently report in maternity services. This is especially crucial given the greater likelihood Autistic mothers face of experiencing both antenatal and postnatal depression (Samuel et al., 2022).

Parenting

Similar to childbirth, Autistic mothering/parenting is an under-researched area; however, the existing research reveals that there are similarly challenging aspects reported. These may include the following:

- Problems in terms of communicating with professionals
- Fear of negative judgement by professionals and others
- Sensory and tactile difficulties when parenting their children
- Lack of, or conversely, overemphasised bodily awareness
- Intense overwhelm and fatigue
- Executive functioning issues
- Isolation and loneliness
- Experience of stigma and dismissive attitude

(Pohl et al., 2020; Hampton et al., 2022).

Several strengths were also noted, including enhanced connection with their Autistic children, lack of concern for the attitudes of others and better understanding of the challenges their Autistic children may experience (Sutcliffe-Khan et al., 2024). For many parents of Autistic children, discovery of their own autism follows their child's diagnosis, and several parents have reported subsequent 'focused interest' on parenting and neurodivergence as a means of gaining knowledge that was invaluable in terms of parenting decisions. Parents also noted a feeling of connection with and acceptance by their children and increased insight into their children's lived experience (Sutcliffe-Khan et al., 2024).

Parents reported that some of the intense demands of parenting could be overwhelming and isolating. The imperative to socialise more and put their children's needs for (for example) socialisation ahead of their own needs (possibly for solitude and quiet) was often perceived as difficult, and parents reported the increased need to 'mask' their autism in social settings (Sutcliff-Khan, 2024; Pohl et. al., 2020). This can be exceedingly tiring and contribute to overall levels of fatigue and overwhelm. Autistic mothers were more likely to find motherhood an isolating experience due to lack of connection and feelings of difference (Pohl et al., 2020). This could be especially profound in settings such as parent groups and when needing to communicate with their children's health professionals and educators (Pohl et al., 2020; Sutcliffe-Khan et al., 2024). Two of the key themes in a study by Thom-Jones et al. (2024) examining Autistic women's experience of motherhood on social media platform Reddit were 'Autistic mothering is different' and 'Autistic mothers need Autistic mothers' (p. 5). Autistic mothers' interactions with other Autistic mothers engendered feelings of normalisation and validation and a sense of solidarity (pp. 5–7). The informal peer support garnered in such settings appears to be invaluable in terms of increasing connection and decreasing loneliness (Thom-Jones et al., 2024).

Together, this existing research on birthing and parenting demonstrates a significant need for the specific needs of birthing people to be further researched and for researchers and policymakers to jointly engage in a process of co-production and design with Autistic birthing people. The 'Report on research, codesign and community engagement to inform the National Roadmap to Improve the Health and Mental Health of Autistic People' (Autism CRC, 2024, p. 9) engaged with a range of stakeholders which included 125 Autistic people, of whom '56 of the parents, carers or guardians of Autistic people also identified as Autistic'. They produced twenty-five recommendations, recommendation twenty of which states:

> Develop and establish national evidence-based standards in pain measurement for Autistic people, considering intersectional experiences and identities across diverse settings such as bedside care, ambulance transport and childbirth, ensuring applicability across all ages and abilities.

While most of the report refers to general healthcare services, several findings and recommendation in this report are highly salient to the maternity context. These include challenges relating to:

- Differences in pain perception and interoception
- Experience of [medical and other] trauma
- Executive functioning difficulties
- Being disbelieved by medical professionals

- Issues around informed consent
- Wishes being ignored
- 'Competing life demands, including parent/carer responsibilities'
- Sensory issues within the healthcare environment

(pp. 30–31)

There is clearly scope to develop this type of consultation and codesign process further in terms of more specific recommendations aimed specifically at birthing people.

Insider research

> Insider research, which occurs through a process of positionality, involves intentionally aligning one's self-interests with one's research.
> Jacobson & Mustafa, 2019

Insider research is research conducted within a social group of which the researcher her/himself is a member (Greene, 2014). It originates in ethnographic field research arising from the disciplines of sociology and anthropology. Insider research is concerned with the researcher's positionality and social location (Green, 2014). As such, the researcher is 'imbricated within the research and possesses an a priori intimate knowledge of the community and its members' (Wilkinson & Kitzinger, 2013, p. 251). While insider research has a long history, its use in autism research is a recent development.

Insider–outsider debate

Kirpitchenko and Voloder (2014) note the existence of a long-standing dichotomy in social science research between insider and outsider research (p. 3). Distinctions of 'Insider-Outsiderness' are predicated on socio-demographic categories of the researcher in comparison to the research group participants – for example, age, gender, ethnicity, social class, sexual orientation, and as of recently, neurodiversity – although as Den Houting et al. (2021, p.148) note, 'participatory autism research is still rare'. Moreover, participatory ADHD research appears absent from the literature. Some scholars argue that insider researchers possess the advantage of inherent knowledge and understanding of a particular group, while outsider researchers possess the necessary distance to question taken-for-granted assumptions (Kirpitchenko & Voloder, 2014).

Influential sociologist Robert Merton (1972) critiqued the notion that only insiders can truly understand the social and cultural nature of a group, arguing that while insider perspectives hold valuable and unique insight, they should not be the only perspectives offered in the research process. The notion of an insider-outsider dichotomy has been strongly contested. Insider status would be better conceptualised as being on a continuum as opposed to a binary and comprises of *total insiders*, who share multiple identities or profound experiences with the community they are studying, and *partial insiders*, who share a sole identity with a certain extent of distance or detachment from the community (Greene, 2014, p. 2).

Benefits

As Merton suggested, neither an insider nor outsider position is superior to the other. That said, there is a strong argument that insider-led research conveys particular benefits. These include:

Knowledge – Insider researchers often do not need to undertake intense orientation processes within the research environment, given that they are usually already familiar with the group characteristics and environment. They also have practical, lived experience of the historical and cultural context of groups and communities.

Access – Access to participants may be easier if the researcher already has contact with groups or individuals, and/or knows the best sites of recruitment.

Ease of interaction – Interactions are more natural, and stereotypical ideas and preconceptions less likely. Non-verbal cues may be perceived by insider researchers, where these are likely to be missed by outsiders. Similarly, any participant attempts at impression management and performativity may be identified more readily.

Relationships – Increased and expedited rapport building based on shared and similar lived experiences (Chavez, 2008; Greene, 2014).

Drawbacks and challenges

Insider positionality may confer disadvantages as well as advantages. Researchers may find forming professional boundaries difficult, which can compromise ethical integrity, compromise the study results and result in overwhelming the researcher in circumstances in which participants have additional expectations of them as a community member. Managing relationships, both professional and personal, may be challenging, and bias may occur in terms of participant selection.

Insider research has been oft-critiqued as being too subjective and bias laden (Chavez, 2008; Greene, 2014; Kirpitchenko, 2014). This is particularly true in disciplines such as psychology which is, as Wilkinson and Kitzinger (2013, p. 251) assert, 'deeply committed to a concept of objectivity that treats insider research as contaminating the production of knowledge'. The same has traditionally applied in sociology, with classical sociologists such as Georg Simmel arguing that the production of knowledge by strangers is more transmissible and superior in terms of scientific rigour (Kirpitchenko & Voloder, 2014). However, as feminist and standpoint scholars have argued, a traditional positivist paradigm seeks to generalise experiences, negating individuality and deep, rich data collection, and 'denying the power of diversity' (Kirpitchenko & Voloder, 2014, p. 5). Moreover, as previously stated, positionality is not binary, nor is it static. Identity cannot be reduced to one sole position; rather, researcher identity must be considered in an intersectional manner that recognises the multiple and diverse intersecting identities of both the insider researcher and the research participants (Couture et al., 2012). Several scholars have discussed their personal experiences of negotiating the insider research experience and have suggested numerous ways in which potential pitfalls may be avoided or minimised (Wilkinson & Kitzinger, 2013; Kirpitchenko & Voloder, 2014).

Participatory research

Participatory research (PR) is research that is carried out with participants as co-producers of knowledge. It is performed *with* them rather than *on* them (Cornwall & Jewkes, 1995). Vaughn and Jacquez (2020) define it as an umbrella term for methods that collaborate with those individuals or groups directly affected by the issue being studied. PR prioritises the co-constructing of research partnerships between researchers and community groups, individuals and other stakeholders not necessarily trained in research methods, engaging in a process of 'sequential reflection and action' (Cornwall & Jewkes, 1995, p. 1667). Participatory research primarily differs from conventional, top-down approaches to research by focusing on issues of power and control, aiming to disrupt hegemonic institutional power structures, and conduct research that is more equitable and democratic, involving participants as coresearchers in the decision-making process (Cornwall & Jewkes, 1995; Vaughn & Jaquez, 2020).

Despite a significant increase in autism research during the last few years, use of participatory models is still rare in terms of autism research (Fletcher-Watson et al., 2019; Den Houting et al., 2021). Den Houting et al. state that despite calls from Autistic academics for more community co-produced research projects, truly equitable research remains uncommon. These are frequently limited to involving community stakeholders in advisory or consultative roles (p. 149). Cornwall and Jewkes (1995) note that there are several 'models' of participatory research ranging from those limited to consulting with communities/individuals through to those based on a Freirean pedagogical model of active participation in creating change. The various levels of participation can be conceptualised using Arnstein's Ladder of Citizen Participation, which ranks participation levels from 'non-participation' (manipulation and therapy) through to 'degrees of tokenism' (informing, consultation, placation) to 'Degrees of citizen power' (partnership, delegated power, citizen control) (Arnstein, 1969).

However, Fletcher-Watson et al. (2019, p. 944) note some critique of this model for, among other issues, its lack of acknowledgement that 'participation itself can be a goal and the process and diversity of experience matter as much as outcome'. They further

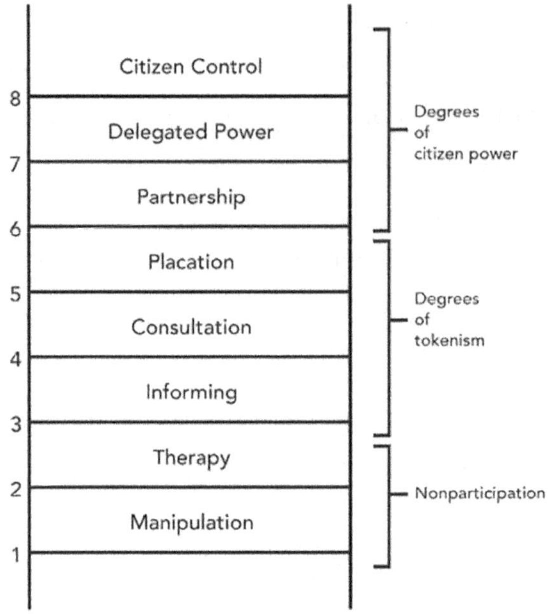

Figure 1: 'Arnstein's ladder'

Note: From A Ladder of Citizen Participation by Arnstein, S, 2019, 216–224, doi:10.1080/01944366908977225.

state that the ladder remains a useful tool for conceptualising power dynamics in autism research, asserting that the majority of research affords either little or merely tokenistic forms of power to participants. Den Houting et al. (2021) note some challenges in terms of conducting participatory research, including the need to balance academic rigour with community participation, the complex nature of managing relationships and greater financial costs; however, they argue that the benefits of community participatory models outweigh its challenges. Similarly, Pellicano et al. (2022) note that not only does PR hold emancipatory power for individuals and communities, but it stands to improve the methodological, scientific and ethics of autism research.

Conclusion: The challenges of a PR PhD

As previously mentioned, incorporating a participatory research approach is something I would have loved to have included in my PhD research; however, systemic and other barriers have precluded this. Nevertheless, I fervently hope that my insider research can include some authentic (if minor) level of co-production (Southby, 2017). Cornwall and Jewkes (1995) argue that rather than methods, researchers' attitudes form the fundamental element of participatory research and that PR is characterised by the location of power (pp. 1667–1668). Researcher reflexivity is an essential component of both insider and participatory approaches (as well as within qualitative research in general). Participatory research is informed by the concerns and values of the community being investigated. As Pillow (cited in Kirpitchenko & Voloder, 2014, p. 5) asserts, being a self-reflexive researcher means not only contributing insider knowledge to research, but also providing 'insight on how this knowledge is produced'. Additionally, the use of autoethnography in terms of incorporating 'self-narrative' or 'personal anecdotes' (p. 10) in one's methodology can be a valuable tool in terms of 'the vulnerability and the humanity of the researcher in relation to a broader social context' (Kirpitchenko & Voloder, 2014).

While it is important to avoid the risk of essentialising insider status to a single homogenous entity, a notion of shared identity can facilitate a sense of belonging, engendering rapport between researcher and participants with the potential to disrupt traditional power relations. Whilst it is crucial to retain strong professional boundaries, I conduct interviews by always considering participants' needs first, ensuring that there are alternatives in terms of meeting place or communication style (e.g. some participants may prefer text-based conversations, others meeting in person, or Zoom); additionally, where appropriate, I like to include discussion of 'what is needed' in terms of healthcare facilities, policy or future research. In my personal experience, many people in the AuDHD space welcome the chance to have their thoughts and opinions noted, and most of my participants have expressed interest in staying informed and connected to the project.

Southby (2017) discusses their PhD research into the experiences of people with a learning disability in football participation in the United Kingdom, noting the 'spectrum' of participatory research in which participation can occur at 'different levels and in unpredictable ways' (p. 130). They reflect upon the challenges of doing participatory research as a research degree student, noting the multiple barriers inherent in the process. While certainly not impossible, practical methodological considerations, such as the structure of a PhD and the proposal process requiring such aspects as the formation of research questions before acceptance into a PhD programme, along with the necessarily rigid ethical procedures, make this difficult. Southby notes that these barriers to doing a participatory PhD may be overcome if the researcher is 'already embedded in the field' in which they wish to research (p. 134). They state that while they would have preferred for their research to be situated further along the participatory continuum, the need to adhere to university protocol to obtain their PhD precluded this; however, they were happy that some level was achieved (p. 139).

The examples discussed throughout this chapter have emphasised the importance of insider, participatory and codesigned research as crucial to understanding the lived experience of neurodivergent individuals. This research, in turn, is vital in terms of informing policy. Recent co-produced research undertaken in partnership with the Australian government informs a report intended to develop a policy 'Roadmap' addressing problematic aspects of healthcare provision for Autistic people in Australia (Autism CRC, 2024). This report reveals similar themes to the existent scholarly research on the lived experiences of neurodivergent mothers. Understanding these challenges and implementing recommendations in a policy context is of crucial importance; however, structural challenges contribute to the scarcity of participatory methodologies in empirical neurodivergence research.

Research methodologies led by neurodivergent researchers are vital to promoting inclusivity and studies conducted through a participatory or co-production lens facilitate meaningful and emancipatory opportunities to amplify the voices of a marginalised community or group. While participatory methods, in particular, present some challenges, the benefits are copious. It would benefit neurodivergent researchers, communities and policymakers if institutional barriers to participatory research were addressed systemically, particularly in terms of funding and the structural processes of PhD and postdoc/early career research. It is hoped that my current PhD research might begin to fill the significant gap in terms of research into the experiences of neurodivergent parents and that future research and policy might address salient areas of need in terms of healthcare and community and social services.

References

Amaze. (2024). *Our language*. https://www.amaze.org.au/about-amaze/our-language/

American Psychiatric Association. (2013). *Diagnostic and statistical manual of mental disorders: DSM-5™* (5th ed.). American Psychiatric Publishing, Inc.

Arnold, S. R., Bruce, G., Weise, J., Mills, C. J., Trollor, J. N., & Coxon, K. (2024). Barriers to healthcare for Australian autistic adults. *Autism: the international journal of research and practice*, 28(2), 301–315. https://doi.org/10.1177/13623613231168444

Arnstein, S. R. (1969). A Ladder Of Citizen Participation. Journal of the American Institute of Planners, 35(4), 216–224. https://doi.org/10.1080/01944366908977225

Australian Bureau of Statistics. (May 2020). *A profile of autism in Australia*, ABS Website, accessed 11 June 2024.

Autism CRC (2024). Report on research, co-design and community engagement to inform the National Roadmap to Improve the Health and Mental Health of Autistic People: Reimagining health services for Autistic people, their families and carers. Autism CRC.

Barnes, C. (2020) in Watson, N., & Vehmas, S. (Eds.). (2020). *Routledge handbook of disability studies* (Second Edition). Routledge.

Charlton, J. I. (1998). *Nothing about us without us: Disability oppression and empowerment*. Univerity of California Press.

Chown, N. (2017). *Understanding and evaluating autism theory*. Jessica Kingsley Publishers.

Chavez, C. (2008). Conceptualizing from the Inside: Advantages, Complications, and Demands on Insider Positionality. *The Qualitative Report*, *13*(3), 474–494.

Cornwall, A., & Jewkes, R. (1995). What is participatory research? *Social Science & Medicine*, *41*(12), 1667–1676. https://doi.org/10.1016/0277-9536(95)00127-S

Couture, A. L., Zaidi, A. U., & Maticka-Tyndale, E. (2012). Reflexive Accounts: An Intersectional Approach to Exploring the Fluidity of Insider/Outsider Status and the Researcher's Impact on Culturally Sensitive Post-Positivist Qualitative Research. *Qualitative Sociology Review*, *8*(1). https://doi.org/10.18778/1733-8077.8.1.05

daVanport, S. (2019). Out of Searching Comes New Vibrance: Edited by Ren Stone. In *Autistic Community and the Neurodiversity Movement: Stories from the Frontline* (pp. 147–154). Singapore: Springer Singapore.

De Broize, M., Evans, K., Whitehouse, A. J. O., Wray, J., Eapen, V., & Urbanowicz, A. (2022). Exploring the Experience of Seeking an Autism Diagnosis as an Adult. *Autism in Adulthood*, *4*(2), 130–140. https://doi.org/10.1089/aut.2021.0028

Den Houting, J., Higgins, J., Isaacs, K., Mahony, J., & Pellicano, E. (2021). 'I'm not just a guinea pig': Academic and community perceptions of participatory autism research. *Autism*, *25*(1), 148–163. https://doi.org/10.1177/1362361320951696

Department of Health and Aged Care. (2024). *National Roadmap to Improve the Health and Mental Health of Autistic People – Consultation draft*. Australian Government. https://www.health.gov.au/resources/publications/autism-roadmap-consultation-draft?language=en

Donovan J. (2020). 'Childbirth experiences of women with autism spectrum disorder in an acute care setting'. *Nurs Womens Health*. 24(3), 165–174. https://doi.org/10.1016/j. nwh.2020.04.001

Fletcher-Watson, S., Adams, J., Brook, K., Charman, T., Crane, L., Cusack, J., ... & Pellicano, E. (2019). Making the future together: Shaping autism research through meaningful participation. *Autism*, *23*(4), 943–953.

Fuller-Thomson, E., Lewis, D. A., & Agbeyaka, S. K. (2016). Attention-deficit/hyperactivity disorder casts a long shadow: Findings from a population-based study of adult women with self-reported ADHD. *Child: Care, Health and Development*, *42*(6), 918–927. https://doi.org/10.1111/cch.12380

Greene. (2014). On the Inside Looking In: Methodological Insights and Challenges in Conducting Qualitative Insider Research. *The Qualitative Report, 19*(29), 1–13.

Hampton, S., Man, J., Allison, C., Aydin, E., Baron-Cohen, S., & Holt, R. (2022). A qualitative exploration of autistic mothers' experiences II: Childbirth and postnatal experiences. *Autism*, *26*(5), 1165–1175. https://doi.org/10.1177/13623613211043701

Hinze, Attwood & Garnett (n.d). Understanding AuDHD Strengths. Attwood & Garnett. https://attwoodandgarnettevents.com/understanding-audhd-strengths/

Garcia, E. (2021). *We're Not Broken: changing the autism conversation*. Harvest.

Garcia, E. (2020). Covering the Politics of Neurodiversity: And Myself. In S.K. Kapp (Ed.). *Autistic Community and the Neurodiversity Movement: Stories from the Frontline.* Springer Singapore. https://doi.org/10.1007/978-981-13-8437-0

Giwa Onaiwu, M. (2019). "A Dream Deferred" No Longer: Backstory of the First Autism and Race Anthology. In Autistic community and the neurodiversity movement: Stories from the frontline (pp. 243–252). Singapore: Springer Singapore.

Jacobson, D., & Mustafa, N. (2019). Social identity map: A reflexivity tool for practicing explicit positionality in critical qualitative research. *International journal of qualitative methods, 18,* 1609406919870075.

Kapp, S. K. (Ed.). (2020). *Autistic Community and the Neurodiversity Movement: Stories from the Frontline*. Springer Singapore. https://doi.org/10.1007/978-981-13-8437-0

Kirpitchenko, L., & Voloder, L. (2014). *Insider Research Method: The Significance of Identities in the Field*. SAGE Publications, Ltd. https://doi.org/10.4135/978144627305014533940

Krewson, C. (2023). Maternal ADHD is associated with postpartum depression risk. *Contemporary OB/GYN*, *68*(8), 17–18.

Lum, M., Garnett, M., & O'Connor, E. (2014). Health communication: A pilot study comparing perceptions of women with and without high functioning autism spectrum disorder. *Research in Autism Spectrum Disorders*, *8*(12), 1713-1721.

Merton, R. K. (1972). Insiders and outsiders: A chapter in the sociology of knowledge. *American journal of sociology*, *78*(1), 9–47.

Mitchell, P., Sheppard, E., & Cassidy, S. (2021). Autism and the double empathy problem: Implications for development and mental health. *British Journal of Developmental Psychology*, *39*(1), 1–18. https://doi.org/10.1111/bjdp.12350

Parliament of New South Wales. (2023). *Select Committee on Birth Trauma. https://www.parliament.nsw.gov.au/committees/listofcommittees/Pages/committee-details.aspx?pk=318*

Pellicano, E., & Den Houting, J. (2022). Annual Research Review: Shifting from 'normal science' to neurodiversity in autism science. *Journal of Child Psychology and Psychiatry*, *63*(4), 381–396. https://doi.org/10.1111/jcpp.13534

Pohl, A. L., Crockford, S. K., Blakemore, M., Allison, C., & Baron-Cohen, S. (2020). A comparative study of autistic and non-autistic women's experience of motherhood. *Molecular Autism*, *11*(1), 3. https://doi.org/10.1186/s13229-019-0304-2

Poulton, A. S., Armstrong, B., & Nanan, R. K. (2018). Perinatal Outcomes of Women Diagnosed with Attention-Deficit/Hyperactivity Disorder: An Australian Population-Based Cohort Study. *CNS Drugs*, *32*(4), 377–386. https://doi.org/10.1007/s40263-018-0505-9

Rasheed Z. (2023). Autism in Australia: Understanding, challenges, and support. *International journal of health sciences*, 17(5), 1–4

Redshaw, M., Malouf, R., Gao, H., & Gray, R. (2013). Women with disability: The experience of maternity care during pregnancy, labour and birth and the postnatal period. *BMC Pregnancy and Childbirth*, *13*(1), 174. https://doi.org/10.1186/1471-2393-13-174

Rosqvist, H. B., Chown, N., & Stenning, A. (2020). *Neurodiversity studies*. Routledge.

Russell, G. (2020). *Critiques of the neurodiversity movement*. Autistic community and the neurodiversity movement, 287.

Samuel P, Yew RY, Hooley M, Hickey M, & Stokes MA. (2022). Sensory challenges experienced by autistic women during pregnancy and childbirth: A systematic review. *Archives of Gynecology and Obstetrics*, *305*(2), 299–311. https://doi.org/10.1007/s00404-021-06109-4

Senate Community Affairs References Committee. (2023). *The Senate Community Affairs References Committee Assessment and support services for people with ADHD*. Parliament of Australia. https://www.aph.gov.au/Parliamentary_Business/Committees/Senate/Community_Affairs/ADHD/Report/Chapter_3_-_Barriers_to_assessment_and_diagnosis

Silberman, S. (2016). *Neurotribes; the legacy of autism and how to think smarter about people who think differently*. (2nd ed.) Allen and Unwin.

Southby, K. (2017). Reflecting on (the challenge of) conducting participatory research as a research-degree student. *Research for All*, *1*(1). https://doi.org/10.18546/RFA.01.1.10

Stace, H. (2011). *Moving beyond love and luck: building right relationships and respecting lived experience in New Zealand autism policy* [Unpublished doctoral dissertation]. Victoria University of Wellington.

Stuart, V. & Kitson-Reynolds, E. (2024). Autistic women's experiences of the antenatal, intrapartum and early postnatal periods. *British Journal of Midwifery*. 34(4), 180–188. https://doi.org/10.12968/bjom.2024.32.4.180

Sutcliffe-Khan, F., Larkin, F., & Hamilton, L. (2024). Parents' and professionals' views on autistic mothers using a participatory research design. *Current Psychology: A Journal for Diverse Perspectives on Diverse Psychological Issues*. https://doi.org/10.1007/s12144-024-05999-2

Sutherland, C. (2024). *When mothers disengage: stories from women who have gone from participants to observers in their autistic child's education* (Doctoral dissertation, Memorial University of Newfoundland).

Talcer, M. C., Duffy, O., & Pedlow, K. (2023). A qualitative exploration into the sensory experiences of autistic mothers. *Journal of Autism and Developmental Disorders*, *53*(2), 834–849.

Thom-Jones, S., Melgaard, I., & Gordon, C. S. (2024). Autistic Women's Experience of Motherhood: A Qualitative Analysis of Reddit. *Journal of Autism and Developmental Disorders, Preprints*, 1–11.

Vaughn, L. M., & Jacquez, F. (2020). Participatory Research Methods – Choice Points in the Research Process. *Journal of Participatory Research Methods*, *1*(1). https://doi.org/10.35844/001c.13244

Walsh, C. J., Rosenberg, S. L., & Hale, E. W. (2022). Obstetric complications in mothers with ADHD. *Frontiers in Reproductive Health*, *4*, 1040824. https://doi.org/10.3389/frph.2022.1040824

Wilkinson, S., & Kitzinger, C. (2013). Representing Our Own Experience: Issues in "Insider" Research. *Psychology of Women Quarterly*, *37*(2), 251–255. https://doi.org/10.1177/0361684313483111

World Health Organization. (2022). *Global report on health equity for persons with disabilities*. World Health Organization.

8
Towards a comprehensive research agenda: Fostering disability inclusion in research and innovation at the University of Queensland

Prof Paul Harpur OAM, Brooke Szucs, Dr Jean McBain, Sarah Brown, Ralph Marszalek, Reshika Chand, and Helen Connick

Introduction

The University of Queensland's (UQ) Champions of Change: Disability Inclusion Research and Innovation Plan (the

Plan) is a disability-inclusive and collaborative research strategy in higher education. The Plan was developed by the Office of the Deputy Vice Chancellor (Research and Innovation) Strategy and Performance Team, specifically the Research Strategy and Policy Team, with the support of Professor Paul Harpur OAM (Medal of the Order of Australia) in his capacity as chair of the UQ Disability Inclusion Group (DIG). Using this Plan, we aim to provide evidence of the value of prioritising disability leadership and collaboration for strategies impacting people with disabilities via a case study of inclusive strategic planning at one of Australia's leading universities.

This chapter detail's the Plan's approach to championing disability inclusion within academic institutions as a case study to highlight to other institutions the benefit of this collaboration process. We emphasize how the approach leads to innovations, addresses barriers to ability equality, promotes diverse representation and actively engages individuals with disabilities in decision-making processes to shape disability policies and research plans. We do this, first, by providing background information on the participation of persons with disabilities within the research process as well as historical approaches that lead to a strategic plan as our response. Second, we outline the methodology used to show the role of people with disabilities within the process, followed by an outline of the outcomes of this process. Last, we analyse and discuss the results, and a demonstration of the relevance of such an approach in future strategies.

The participatory dynamic

The UNCRPD has introduced a transformative participatory framework that mandates States and other actors engage and resource persons with disabilities to be involved in developing, implementing and monitoring policies affecting their community (Harpur & Stein, 2022). Early in its formulation, the drafters of the CRPD recognized the benefit of involving persons with disabilities in policy discussions that impact them, with the Chair of the Ad Hoc Committee granting Disabled Persons Organizations participant status in the drafting process (Harpur & Stein, 2022). States' parties involved in this process recognised the importance of having disability representatives present and embedded this participatory approach in the convention, notably in Articles 4(3) and 33(3) (United Nations, 2018).

These articles mandate that persons with disabilities and their representative bodies be empowered to actively participate in the CRPD's implementation. The CRPD Committee, responsible for monitoring the convention, elaborates on this participatory requirement in its General Comment #7 providing detailed guidelines for how States and other actors must realize the participatory dynamic and enact 'nothing about us without us' (United Nations, 2018).

Central to the participatory dynamic is the distinction between mere consultation, which involves seeking information towards the end of a process, and codesign or co-creation, which actualizes participation by including and equipping persons with disabilities and their representative bodies throughout the entire process – from design and drafting to implementation and monitoring of disability inclusion initiatives (Harpur & Stein, 2022). Achieving this participatory framework demands substantial efforts from States and other stakeholders to build capacity and effectively implement it. This is crucial in realizing the transformative potential of the CRPD in advancing disability rights and ensuring a paradigm shift towards inclusive human rights practices that centre those directly impacted.

Status of disability research

Research on persons with disabilities has often failed to embrace the participatory dynamic. Instead, disability-related research has been dominated by non-disabled persons from a medical lens, excluding the possibility of full participation and representation of the disability community.

Within the main research institutions of Australia (our universities), there is a shortage of disability representation within university executive positions (Harpur & Szucs, 2023). Although there are many reasons why those with non-apparent disabilities may be in such roles and not wish to disclose, the majority of researcher leaders present as non-disabled (Yerbury & Yerbury, 2021). There is also limited research into the status of higher degree by research students in the Australian and international context, although what does exist indicates the lack of support and difficulties faced by these students (Spier & Natalier, 2023). This is despite PhD students being the pipeline for our future research workforce. Other university-specific barriers – access to completing education – also disproportionately impact this student group, such as poor university policies on access to digital books for the print disabled (Harpur & Loudoun, 2011). We can also make the assumption that this under-represented group follows many of the struggles of other minorities in higher education such as lower enrolment and success rates (Brownlow et al., 2023). We can further contextualise this with the participation rates of undergraduate students with disabilities in Australian universities, which is currently reported to be at 9.4%, despite the population of Australians with disabilities estimated to be at 18% (Australian Institute of Health and Welfare, 2022, 2024).

With the pipeline for student to academic already demonstrating challenges, there are further barriers to those who do become academics with disabilities. As well as the continuation of issues present during the student life cycle, such as access to digital resources necessary for academia, new issues emerge (Harpur, 2017). These challenges include discrimination and loss of opportunity for disclosing a disability in the workplace as well as more logistical challenges (Thom-Jones, 2022; Yerbury & Yerbury, 2021). For example, an Australian academic is often expected to travel for work, including activities essential for career advancement such as conferences (Pegg et al., 2021). However, this attracts significant extra costs of time, money and energy for academics with disabilities compared with those without. For example, they may need to rely on a guide, need to bring their personal carer or book a more expensive hotel room with the necessary facilities (Karl et al., 2022). With the added stress and financial pressure from these considerations, there are many who opt out, further impacting their careers (Pegg et al., 2021). Although some funding exists from UQ to support their academics traveling for work, this is far from the norm (Workplace Diversity and Inclusion, 2022). All of these factors, and more, cumulate in an Australian academic landscape that rarely features those with disabilities, especially in leadership positions (Harpur & Szucs, 2023).

A research landscape dominated by non-disabled people does not fulfil the expectations led by the CRPD, which requires the full participation of persons with disabilities in all areas of life concerning them (Harpur & Stein, 2022; United Nations, 2018). Furthermore, there is historical advocacy for a greater role of researchers with a disability to improve academic outcomes (Stone & Priestley, 1996). Stone and Priestley (1996) highlighted the tendency for research by non-disabled researchers to be ableist and unethical, such as by prioritising the views of practitioners treating disabilities above the individuals. Oliver (1992) and Kitchin (2000) elaborate how research outputs do not represent the researched community and can further alienate and disempower the disability community. Negative views of persons with disabilities continue, with such viewpoints being illustrated by a 2024 article calling homeless people with personality disorders 'super difficult patients', again highlighting the perspective of the practitioner over the disabled individual (Henriques-Calado & Gama Marques, 2024).

Much of this previous criticism comes from the fact that many practitioners and disability researchers rely on the medical model of disability. This model frames disability as a deficit that needs to be treated and remedied, and those with disabilities being discounted citizens (Adame, 2014). Indeed, there is a strong perception that this model is linked to eugenics, institutionalisation and segregation of disabled people (Adame, 2014; Kitchin, 2000). Meanwhile, research from disability advocates and disabled people embraces the social model of disability, which instead focuses on strengths and outside factors that disable a person and highlights 'nothing about us without us' (Inckle et al., 2023).

The result of the research landscape being dominated by the medical model and non-disabled researchers was a long-standing culture where those with disabilities have felt used, irrelevant and overall unhelpful to improving the lives of their communities (Inckle et al., 2023; Oliver, 1992). Indeed, the general sentiment from those with disabilities has been consistently negative in relation to their capacity to enact meaningful social change as well as further entrenching power dynamics (Kitchin, 2000; Oliver, 1992; Stone & Priestley, 1996).

Change was needed to improve research outcomes and participation for the disability community, to overcome the fact that 'research has been experienced as exploitative, oppressive and unrepresentative, and many disabled people are suspicious of able-bodied researchers' (Inckle et al., 2023).

Strategies as a response

A well-defined university strategy can contribute to positive change in research culture by providing a structured framework for actions, centred around a principles-based ambition for change. This framework typically includes clear objectives, measurable KPIs (key performance indicators), and actionable items that guide researchers and stakeholders towards impactful outcomes. It fosters accountability among all involved parties, ensuring that efforts are directed towards achieving tangible results in research. Additionally, a strategic approach helps in aligning resources effectively, maximizing collaboration opportunities and ultimately advancing the field with meaningful contributions and innovations. As a university strategy is an expression of top-down priorities and values, this format is especially pertinent to improving outcomes for minorities in research, who may not be best positioned within university structures to enact change.

To illustrate, other marginalised communities within higher education and research participation have addressed similar issues of collaboration and meaningful engagement via strategies. For example, the peak body Universities Australia, as part of its Indigenous Strategy 2017–2020, committed all thirty-nine-member universities to 'have Indigenous Research Strategies in place' (Universities Australia, 2017). The University of Queensland fulfilled this commitment with the Aboriginal and Torres Strait Islander Research and Innovation Strategy (2021–2025), which explicitly follows the same ethos of inclusion, self-determination and centring of First Nations voices (The University of Queensland, 2021). The inclusive and collaborative model for this strategy lent itself to success, with UQ leading the first awarded Indigenous-led Australian Research Council Centre of Excellence in 2022, with AUD 35 million of funding over 7 years (Australian Research Council, 2022). Other successes included access to AUD 400,000 in research funding, growth in Aboriginal and Torres Strait Islander HDR enrolments, improved access to data commons to improve Indigenous research capacity and the hosting of Indigenous Knowledge Centre researchers to improve collaboration and access (The University of Queensland, 2022).

The Plan as a response

UQ seeks to become a disability champion of change and has engaged in several university-wide initiatives to create a more inclusive society. As part of this effort to champion inclusion, UQ is committed to empower and resource a co-creation process to develop a Champions of Change: Disability Inclusion and Research Innovation Plan (the Plan) as one key aspect of this change agenda. The Plan followed the notion of achieving excellence in disability research centres on having individuals with disabilities in a leadership position throughout the entire research process, from the initial project stages to the implementation and influence of findings. This section details how the development of the Plan sought to uphold the fundamental principle of inclusion 'nothing about us without us' by engaging those with disabilities in the decision-making process.

The Plan not only leverages significant events like the 2032 Olympics and Paralympics but also capitalizes on the university's expanding expertise in intersectionality. By explicitly targeting research by people with disabilities, disability research itself, support for professional staff working with researchers with disabilities and engagement with end users of disability research, the Plan covers a broad spectrum of opportunities for promoting inclusion and accessibility. This comprehensive approach demonstrates a nuanced understanding of disability inclusion within the research and innovation context, ensuring that diverse perspectives are integrated into every facet of the university's research endeavours.

The concept of a university-wide disability inclusion research plan was initially discussed during the preparation of the University of Queensland Disability Action Plan 2018–2021 (UQ DAP). Rather than creating a comprehensive plan, Clause 4.6 of this document committed the university to promoting and supporting research aimed at fostering a disability-inclusive environment. Academic and operational researchers at UQ utilized this strategic commitment to develop a research agenda that contributed to the university's goals of enhancing disability inclusion. One aspect of this research agenda was resourcing academic and professional staff to collaborate on co-creating policy solutions for the university, while at the same time enabling academics to use this process to produce academic outputs (Karl et al., 2022). The success of disability-related research laid the groundwork for shaping the current DAP (2023–2025), which includes a commitment by UQ to develop a Disability Inclusion Research and Innovation Plan.

The creation of the Disability Inclusion Research and Innovation Plan was guided by the ethos and principles of the CRPD, already apparent in the process for creating the DAP (The University of Queensland, 2023b). This precedent would continue moving forward into leadership and responsibility of the project, as the strategy's oversight lies with the chair of the DIG, who themselves live with a disability.

The creation of the Plan relied on extensive consultations with members of the disability community. By centring the voices and experiences of individuals with disabilities in the Plan's development, it ensures that the resulting initiatives are not only sensitive to their needs but also reflective of their lived realities. Such inclusivity not only promotes equity but also leads to innovations and enhances the effectiveness and relevance of the Plan in addressing the diverse challenges faced by the disability community for research inclusion within our institution. All of this, in consideration with the previously mentioned challenges with disability research, clearly demonstrated a need for further action in this area.

The rest of this chapter details the collaboration and highlights the outputs of such an approach.

Methodology

Data collection and collaboration

The scope of the Plan was initially defined after the project team (the Research Strategy and Policy Team) conducted a thorough review of the existing literature, including peer-reviewed and grey literature, focusing on 'Disability Inclusion Research Plans'. Specifically, this desktop review encompassed disability strategies, action plans, agendas and guidelines from Australian universities, state and federal governments and NGOs (non-governmental organisations). The goal was to determine the parameters and objectives that the Plan should aim to encompass. Additionally, the Plan's objectives were aligned with the structure and goals outlined in the UQ Research Roadmap, a document which guides the University's overall research endeavour (The University of Queensland, n.d.).

The development of the Plan was informed by a multistage consultation and drafting approach across the University over one year. The first part of the consultation was in two stages: an online survey and focus groups. Input and feedback as to the potential vision, values, and ambitions for the Plan were gathered via survey, while more in-depth opinions and ideas from stakeholders were gathered via the focus groups to guide development of the Plan.

Ethics was provided under UQ Ethics number 2023/HE001520.

Survey

A total of sixty-eight participants took part in the online survey, comprising staff and HDR students. Among them, thirty-one voluntarily disclosed a disability.

The survey was designed to comprehensively assess disability inclusion research and innovation at UQ through a series of focused questions. It sought to understand the current state of disability inclusion efforts, identifying key areas for improvement and information gaps necessary to support researchers who live with a disability. Additionally, the survey aimed to envision future aspirations for UQ in disability research and sought opinions on how the university can emerge as a leader in this field at local, national and global levels. 'Vision' questions explored stakeholders' perspectives on UQ's role in enabling and facilitating disability-related research by staff and students, while 'values' questions aimed to investigate individual viewpoints on what disability inclusion means and how UQ should prioritize its efforts in this area.

Focus groups

In total, twenty-seven participants consisting of staff, HDR students and persons with disabilities took part in six focus groups. These sessions involved a total of fifty participant instances, as some individuals signed up for and attended more than one focus group because each session had a different topic. On average, each participant engaged in just under two focus groups, highlighting their active involvement and contribution across multiple sessions. This diverse participation ensured that comprehensive perspectives were gathered and considered in the discussions and outcomes of the focus groups.

The focus groups at UQ were structured around five distinct topics aimed at comprehensively addressing various facets of disability research and support within the university. These topics were: supporting researchers with disabilities; assessing UQ's capabilities and achievements in disability research; examining research impact and engagement with end users; exploring partnerships for advancing disability research initiatives; and identifying training and development needs for researchers and those working in research support and administration. A seventh session was held in-person with the UQ Disability Community of Practice and asked participants to express their opinions on the items outlined above. A group discussion was facilitated by the project team and asked participants to collaborate on their responses to the discussion items.

Note on disclosure: Members of the focus groups were not asked for their disability status, as disclosure can be a complicated topic (Yerbury & Yerbury, 2021). However, the attendees were active members of the disability community, and many disclosed their disability voluntarily as part of their responses.

Data analysis

Data analysis was performed by the Strategy and Policy Team. The qualitative output of the sources was collated and de-identified. A thematic analysis was then conducted to create the draft action items for a 2024–2026 Action Plan, the key outcome-focused component of the larger Plan. Three authors manually processed and analysed the data to create the key interest areas. These were validated by other members of the team. Measures, responsibilities and delivery timeframes were then also drafted to accompany the key action items.

Creating the Plan

The Plan was developed by the Strategy and Policy Team through extensive engagement and liaison with owners of draft action items, ensuring each was achievable, appropriate and fit for purpose. Following this, the consultation draft was disseminated across the university and invited final feedback and comments to refine and finalize the plan; this activity also served as the third consultative exercise. The Plan currently awaits executive final approvals and will go to the Research and Ethics Committee for endorsement. Publication of the final Plan is scheduled for September 2024.

Results

The above participatory approach resulted in consistent participant feedback centring on four domains: Researchers and Research Culture, Research and Innovation Enabling Capabilities, Research Investment and Cross-Disciplinary Collaboration, and Research Infrastructure, Systems and Precincts. These domains align with the UQ Research Roadmap, which will support operationalization of the Plan through the university's annual planning and reporting processes.

Researchers and research culture

There was a high level of interest in the experiences of HDR students as future research leaders and as direct participants.

Participants identified several challenges within the HDR context, including a perceived lack of support resources directed towards HDR students compared to undergraduate students. One survey respondent expressed this as:

> My disability advisor didn't know how to set up an SAP [Student Access Plan] for me because it's mainly used for undergraduates. The overall structure of the SAPs for HDRs needs to be thought through.

Financial hardships were highlighted, particularly concerning the need for stipends and scholarships tailored to support students managing disabilities. The survey respondents emphasized the necessity of financial assistance to cover disability-related costs for HDR students designed to alleviate the financial burdens associated with pursuing higher education for students with disabilities. As expressed by a focus group participant:

> … the lack of HDR students identifying with a disability, particularly those [with disabilities] that are expensive… Because we can't afford to support ourselves on a stipend. And so, if you want to encourage people with a disability to participate in research and keep them there, they have to be able to afford to get through it, right?

Additionally, participants emphasized the need for comprehensive training programmes for academic advisors of HDR students (the local term for PhD supervisors) to better understand and utilize available support systems for their students. They also expressed concerns about research environments perceived as unwelcoming and ableist within higher education.

Participants also advocated for inclusive training initiatives aimed at promoting disability awareness and combating ableism among both staff and students. These insights underscore the participants' collective push for systemic improvements to ensure equitable access and support within academic and research environments for researchers managing disabilities. As one focus group participant expressed:

> …training for supervisors on how to manage and be more open and accepting of people with disability. In

> my personal experience I've had similar situations of questioning whether you're really sick. [That] You look fine today.

For more general researcher improvement, participants expressed that funds dedicated to researchers with disabilities would allow for these individuals to gain a higher researcher profile in line with their opportunity, while also cementing UQ as a disability research leader.

Research and innovation enabling capabilities

Participants emphasized the critical need for trust building within the disability community, highlighting the positive impact of having disabled individuals in leadership roles within research endeavours. This leadership representation was seen as essential for ensuring that research outcomes are relevant and trusted by those they aim to benefit.

There was a shared sentiment among participants regarding the necessity to manage expectations realistically in disability research. They noted how promising research outcomes that might be hindered by funding constraints, governmental policies, and other factors without explaining this possibility to participants damaged trust. As one focus group participant explained:

> … building trust with the disability community, it's hard to maintain because if you're working with the university or with government or with, a big business. And then you're also working with community or go between. And essentially the end of the day, a workable solution

is probably going to be something that neither side will be happy with...

Participants also advocated for disseminating research findings beyond traditional academic journals to more accessible formats such as YouTube videos, which can effectively showcase tangible results to the broader community. They also linked this to adding further value to researchers with disabilities, who may find such outputs more accessible and relevant than traditional research outputs.

Collaboration with local communities and organizations was identified as pivotal in disability inclusion research. Engaging external stakeholders was viewed as crucial for developing practical solutions and promoting positive social change. Participants expressed that such a collaborative approach would reflect UQ's commitment to responsible and engaged research that directly serves and involves the community.

Specifically, participants proposed the establishment of a pre-award research funding system aimed at consulting with individuals with lived experiences of disabilities, saying that this initiative would facilitate meaningful partnerships between UQ researchers and the disability community, ensuring that research efforts are inclusive and address real-world needs effectively.

Research investment and cross-disciplinary collaboration

Participants in the discussion emphasized UQ's potential to spearhead linkage partnerships, advocating for multidisciplinary approaches that integrate disability into diverse realms of research. They proposed a requirement for disability co-leadership or substantial collaboration to access external funding, aiming to ensure research projects directly address the needs of the disability community and avoid tokenism. Highlighting UQ's Paralympics Centre of Excellence, participants saw an opportunity not only to advance medical and sports research but also to champion the social model of disability and empower researchers with a disability (The University of Queensland, 2023a).

Additionally, there was a strong call for dedicated funding streams supporting research by individuals with disabilities, coupled with the creation of an online platform to consolidate and navigate UQ's disability research efforts. These proposed initiatives reflect a collective vision to enhance UQ's leadership in inclusive research practices, leveraging its resources to foster impactful collaborations and drive meaningful advancements in disability studies and beyond.

Research infrastructure, systems and precincts

Participants highlighted several challenges they encountered in accessing various aspects of their university experience. These difficulties encompassed physical access barriers, limitations in accessing research systems and resources and ethical concerns in consulting the disability community. For instance, one HDR survey respondent cited the struggle of needing remote access to digital resources due to physical barriers preventing them from reaching the library and policies preventing access to digital books:

> It makes life more difficult for the student with a disability, especially when trying to attain physical library books.

Ethics procedures were also criticized for their complexity, discouraging some from engaging in initial consultations with the disability community.

Additionally, there was a pressing need expressed for improved access to necessary equipment to support individuals with disabilities. Participants called for greater flexibility in work arrangements and the creation of inclusive and accessible buildings. For example, labs were consistently identified as areas requiring improvements in accessibility infrastructure. These concerns underscored the participants' advocacy for systemic changes to enhance inclusivity and ensure equitable access to educational resources and opportunities within the university environment.

The results of the research directly informed the key focus areas of the Plan (further examined in the discussion).

Discussion and implications for research agenda.

Reflecting on how the Plan serves as a case study justifying the prioritization of disability-inclusive research strategies, this discussion explores the potential implications for the broader research agenda in higher education institutions worldwide.

Resulting actions from the Plan

The Plan created from this collaborative process reflects the themes expressed by the participants and outlined in the literature to address the strategic and operational demands of the university.

Researchers and research culture

This focus area states that UQ will empower staff and student researchers with disabilities by fostering an environment of excellence and inclusion. UQ pledges to support and champion their work, enabling them to create lasting impacts and lead in knowledge dissemination. Additionally, UQ plans to enhance cross-institutional capacity for high-quality disability inclusion research through professional development and best practice guidance initiatives.

Examples of specific deliverables in the Action Plan are:

Action: Improve our capacity to support HDR candidates living with disability.

Measure: Review HDR scholarships policy to ensure that candidates living with disability can access support required for completion.

This commitment resonates with the community's viewpoint outlining the significance of including researchers with disabilities. The aforementioned historical exclusion of individuals with disabilities from participating as researchers means that it is crucial to prioritize the advancement of researchers with disabilities to tackle this issue effectively (Harpur & Szucs, 2023; Stone & Priestley, 1996). This point aligns with the findings of other universities within Australia, such as La Trobe University that offers a Flexible Research Scholarship which funds extensions to doctoral and research masters candidates (La Trobe University, 2023):

Action: Improve support for researchers with disability in evidencing research achievements in grants applications.

Measure: Continue to skill research office staff who are providing guidance on describing and evidencing research performance relative to opportunity.

This action aligns with community needs by expanding access to opportunities that may otherwise be limited. This is particularly significant for individuals who face barriers such as travel requirements to access traditional or existing resources, which are highly valued on grant applications (Karl et al., 2022; Pegg et al., 2021).

Research and innovation enabling capabilities

UQ is dedicated to fostering excellence in disability inclusion research and to leveraging researchers' expertise to develop and apply knowledge, especially to support disability research and involve researchers with disabilities in engaging with end users, aiming for collaborative partnerships and practical outcomes.

Action: Promote best practice in codesign and co-production of knowledge.

Measure: Determine needs and, where required, provide opportunities or resources for members of UQ Human Research Ethics Committees to develop their skills in assessing disability inclusion, codesign and/or co-production principles in research ethics applications.

As the UQ ethics process already requires researchers to properly articulate the expectations and purpose of their research in a general manner, a specific understanding of how this impacts the disability community will be well placed to create a lasting change. This move aims at improving how people with disabilities experience participation in research and to alleviate concerns associated with the medical model and non-disabled researchers (Inckle et al., 2023; Kitchin, 2000; Oliver, 1992). The importance of the principles of codesign and co-production will further work to limit the sense that the research is irrelevant or not impactful to the communities in question.

Research investment and cross-disciplinary collaboration

This focus area of the Plan highlights the importance of the university strengthening its disability research capability through interdisciplinary collaboration internally and with external partners. It aims to foster long-term engagement across the organization to advance disability research and innovation, particularly in relation to opportunities emerging from Brisbane's hosting of the 2032 Olympics and Paralympics:

Action: Increase profile of disability research for internal and external stakeholders.

Measure: Develop a collection of research impact stories profiling examples of codesign and co-production in disability inclusion research on the research news website.

This action and measure will emphasise the importance of how involving persons with disabilities in research processes leads to meaningful outcomes that benefit the community. The increased profile of disability research will also encourage greater participation and engender increased trust from key stakeholders:

Action: Target research partnerships aligned with the Brisbane 2032 agenda.

Measure: Build an institutional framework to capitalise on opportunities aligned with the 2032 Olympics and Paralympics, targeting partnerships for research engagement and impact.

This strategic approach utilizes the global spotlight on the Brisbane Olympics to plan for impactful research collaborations that advance disability inclusion initiatives locally and globally. This will also hopefully serve to improve the funding available to academics with disabilities and improve their access to professional development, an issue highlighted frequently by participants (Karl et al., 2022; Pegg et al., 2021).

Research infrastructure, systems and precincts

In response to the system deficits raised by participants, the Plan will maximize opportunities to ensure that top-tier research infrastructure and capabilities are accessible, applying universal design principles to both physical infrastructure and digital research management systems:

Action: Extend accessibility of research infrastructure.

Measure: Review activities and, where relevant, promote availability of remote access and/or remote operation of UQ owned, managed or hosted research infrastructure.

This action and measure directly address the need for those within the university to be able to access tools and resources needed for their research, education and career progression (as highlighted earlier); for example, ensuring the university community has access to research platforms in digital form for the print-disabled (Harpur, 2017).

Other innovations

Other factors that make this Plan so innovative include the importance placed on real issues that reflect the values of the disability community. One such factor is the emphasis on the social model of disability, which aligns with the disability community's preference (Inckle et al., 2023).

Areas outside the remit of the Plan

The Plan addresses a crucial aspect of the research pipeline, focusing specifically on current research talent. The alignment of the DIG Chair, in both overseeing the Plan and supporting the DAP with respect to teaching, ensures coherent strategic approach to the uplift of disability inclusion research and facilitates achievable capacity building.

While the Plan is comprehensive, it does have limitations in its design. For example, it does not extend to the undergraduate-to-graduate pipeline. Even though these students are captured by existing student supports as well as referenced in the UQ's DAP, further work on developing the research talent of students with disabilities is planned once recent Universities Accord reforms have been finalised. As a result, potential researchers with disabilities may not receive support until later stages, possibly excluding, at an early stage, a portion of academic and research talent from this potential career pathway. However, this limitation underscores the Plan's focus on current research talent rather than evidencing a shortfall in consulting and involving people with disabilities.

Next steps

The Plan incorporates robust governance and accountability measures to guarantee the achievement of key objectives and actions. This includes the establishment of a detailed implementation plan and an annual reporting process to include comprehensive key performance metrics.

Looking ahead, the Plan will be renewed for the 2027–2029 and 2030–2032 iterations, further enhancing its foundational values and extending these initiatives even further. This iterative approach aims to continually improve and adapt to the evolving needs of the disability research community.

Each of these future ambitions for the Plan will involve collaboration and leadership with people with disabilities, such as the inclusion of the UQ DIG on overseeing the implementation plans and annual reports. This will ensure the continuing relevance of the Plan to the disability community across the university and towards meeting the values prescribed by the Plan.

Wider applications

While this case study shows the situation within the university context, universities are organisations that operate much like others in a wider range of industries. For example, this same method of iterative consultation and disability-led oversight for research has relevance for the development of plans and policies in other organisational contexts. This includes disability hiring, recruitment and support strategies for those who wish to better connect with their clients, attract new staff/students or improve employee outcomes.

This consultative and inclusive method can also be applied for smaller scale initiatives, such as reviews of programmes or products, performance reviews or policy and programme development for organisations. Although the specifics may differ, the importance the Plan places on reflecting current and relevant issues to the disability community shows the value to the organisation and community on such an approach.

Conclusion

Throughout this chapter, we have explained the process needed to meaningfully engage the disability community in the development of a research plan that enables researchers, participants and students with a disability to achieve their full potential. This has resulted in a plan that clearly aligns with many of the main issues with disability research participation and conduct, evident within the wider academic literature and the lived experiences of participants and the expectations of the CRPD.

These main themes of the Plan were: Researchers and Research Culture, Research and Innovation Enabling Capabilities, Research Investment and Cross-disciplinary Collaboration and Research Infrastructure, Systems and Precincts. Addressing disability inclusion across each of these focus areas will significantly improve UQ's disability research capacity as well as researcher development, in a way that will further support persons with disabilities' engagement in society. Further research may evaluate the impacts of such a plan after implementation. However, the current relevance of the Plan clearly aligns with the needs of the community as presented in academic literature and our own data collection.

For too long, disability research has been a lot about us, without us. Even worse, about us, in a way that looks down on us or judges us. When large research institutions, or any institution at all, take the opportunity to reflect and actively work towards inclusion, we can bypass 'nothing about us without us' and realise the ideal of 'nothing about us, unless it is led by us'.

References

Adame, A. L. (2014). "There Needs to be a Place in Society for Madness": The Psychiatric Survivor Movement and New Directions in Mental Health Care. *Journal of Humanistic Psychology*, *54*(4), 456–475. https://doi.org/10.1177/0022167813510207

Australian Institute of Health and Welfare. (2022). *People with disability in Australia*. Australian Government. https://www.aihw.gov.au/reports/disability/people-with-disability-in-australia/contents/people-with-disability/prevalence-of-disability

Australian Institute of Health and Welfare. (2024). *People with disability in Australia: Engagement in Education*. Australian Government. https://www.aihw.gov.au/reports/disability/people-with-disability-in-australia/contents/education-and-skills/engagement-in-education

Australian Research Council. (2022). *ARC Centre of Excellence for Indigenous Futures*. Australian Government. https://www.arc.gov.au/funding-research/discovery-linkage/linkage-program/arc-centres-excellence/arc-centre-excellence-indigenous-futures

Brownlow, C., Eacersall, D. C., Martin, N., & Parsons-Smith, R. (2023). The higher degree research student experience in Australian universities: a systematic literature review. *Higher Education Research*

& Development, *42*(7), 1608–1623. https://doi.org/10.1080/07294360.2023.2183939

Harpur, P. (2017). *Discrimination, Copyright and Equality: Opening the e-Book for the Print-Disabled*. Cambridge University Press. https://doi.org/https://doi.org/10.1017/9781316340516

Harpur, P., & Loudoun, R. (2011). The barrier of the written word: analysing universities' policies to students with print disabilities. *Journal of Higher Education Policy and Management, 33*(2), 153–167. https://doi.org/10.1080/1360080X.2011.550088

Harpur, P., & Stein, M. A. (2022). The Convention on the Rights of Persons With Disabilities as a Global Tipping Point for the Participation of Persons With Disabilities. *The Oxford Encyclopedia of Human Rights*. Oxford University Press. https://doi.org/10.1093/acrefore/9780190228637.013.245

Harpur, P., & Szucs, B. (2023). Using the new disability human rights paradigm to create higher education leadership opportunities. *International Journal of Discrimination and the Law*, *23*(1–2), 144–162. https://doi.org/10.1177/13582291231169668

Henriques-Calado, J., & Gama Marques, J. (2024). Homeless people: a review of personality disorders. *Front Psychiatry*, *15*. https://doi.org/10.3389/fpsyt.2024.1362723

Inckle, K., Brighton, J., & Sparkes, A. C. (2023). Who is "Us" in "Nothing About Us Without US"? Rethinking the Politics of Disability Research. *Disability Studies Quarterly 42*(3–4). https://dsq-sds.org/index.php/dsq/article/view/7947/7859

Karl, M., Pegg, S., & Harpur, P. (2022). Exploring constraints in business travel for disabled workers: An ecological systems perspective. *Disability & Society*, *3,* 1–24. https://doi.org/10.1080/09687599.2022.2088333

Kitchin, R. (2000). The Researched Opinions on Research: Disabled people and disability research. *Disability & Society*, *15*(1), 25–47. https://doi.org/10.1080/09687590025757

La Trobe University. (2023). *La Trobe Flexible Research Scholarship*. https://www.latrobe.edu.au/study/scholarships/other/la-trobe-flexible-research-scholarship-flex-candidates-with-disabilities#:~:text=This%20scholarship%20provides%20individually%20tailored,associated%20with%20having%20a%20disability

Oliver, M. (1992). Changing the Social Relations of Research Production? *Disability, Handicap & Society*, *7*(2), 101–114. https://doi.org/10.1080/02674649266780141

Pegg, S., Karl, M., & Harpur, P. (2021). Negotiating work-based travel for people with disabilities. *Current Issues in Tourism*, *24*(14), 1945–1951. https://doi.org/10.1080/13683500.2020.1801605

Spier, J., & Natalier, K. (2023). Reasonable adjustments? Disabled research higher degree students' strategies for managing their candidature in an Australian university. *Disability & Society*, *38*(8), 1365–1386. https://doi.org/10.1080/09687599.2021.1997718

Stone, E., & Priestley, M. (1996). Parasites, Pawns and Partners: Disability Research and the Role of Non-Disabled Researchers. *The British Journal of Sociology*, *47*(4), 699–716. https://doi.org/10.2307/591081

The University of Queensland. (2021). *The University of Queensland Aboriginal and Torres Strait Islander Research and Innovation Strategy 2021 - 2025*. https://research-support.uq.edu.au/files/39775/20210223%20UQ%20Aboriginal%20and%20Torres%20Strait%20Islander%20Research%20and%20Innovation%20Strategy%202021-2025.pdf

The University of Queensland. (2022). *Aboriginal and Torres Strait Islander Research and Innovation Strategy Annual Report 2022*. https://research-support.uq.edu.au/files/80583/Aboriginal%20and%20Torres%20Strait%20Islander%20Research%20and%20Innovation%20Strategy%20Annual%20Report%202022_online.pdf

The University of Queensland. (2023a). *Brisbane on track to be Australia's home of Paralympic sport.* https://stories.uq.edu.au/news/2023/brisbane-on-track-to-be-australias-home-of-paralympic-sport/index.html

The University of Queensland. (2023b). *Disability Action Plan 2023–2025.* https://staff.uq.edu.au/files/110634/Disability%20Action%20Plan%20V8b.pdf

The University of Queensland. (n.d.). *Research Roadmap.* https://www.uq.edu.au/research/research-roadmap

Thom-Jones, S. (2022). *Growing into Autism.* Melbourne University Press.

United Nations. (2018). *General comment No.7 on Article 4.3 and 33.3 - the participation of persons with disabilities in the implementation and monitoring of the Convention.* https://www.ohchr.org/en/documents/general-comments-and-recommendations/general-comment-no7-article-43-and-333-participation

Universities Australia. (2017). *Universities Australia Indigenous Strategy 2017–2020.* https://universitiesaustralia.edu.au/wp-content/uploads/2019/06/Indigenous-Strategy-v16-1.pdf

Workplace Diversity and Inclusion. (2022). *Staff with Disability Travel Support Fund - Procedural Guidance.* University of Queensland. https://staff.uq.edu.au/files/32546/staff-with-disability-travel-fund.pdf

Yerbury, J. J., & Yerbury, R. M. (2021). Disabled in academia: to be or not to be, that is the question. *Trends in Neurosciences, 44*(7), 507–509. https://doi.org/https://doi.org/10.1016/j.tins.2021.04.004

Discussion questions

1. What are some of the challenges in defining what counts as lived experience of disability?
2. Why is it important to incorporate perspectives which are informed by lived experience of disability codevelopment of policies, for example, those relating to restrictive practices, older persons with dual sensory impairment and health experiences in rural locations. Describe the potential for policymakers to address the pressing policy issue of information deprivation and the subsequent social and economic exclusion of people with disability.
3. What did you learn about the current gaps in Australian disability policy concerning meeting the needs of older people living with dual sensory impairment? How can these be best addressed?
4. Why is codesigned and co-produced research important for informing evidence-based disability policy directions?
5. What are some of the fundamental barriers to inclusion that are experienced by Australian academics with disability?

Recommended further reading

Dew, A., Plumb, J., Gallego, G., Garbellini, S., Imms, C., Darcy, S., McVilly, K., Hemsley, B., O'Donovan, M.A. and Smith-Merry, J., 2022. Setting an agenda for disability research in Australia: synthesis and refinement.

Harpur, P. and Szucs, B., 2023. Using the new disability human rights paradigm to create higher education leadership opportunities. *International Journal of Discrimination and the Law*, *23*(1–2), pp.144–162.

Harpur, P., Szucs, B. and Willox, D., 2023. Strategic and policy responses to intersectionality in higher education. *Journal of Higher Education Policy and Management*, *45*(1), pp.19–35.

Mellifont, D., Watharow, A., Daniels-Mayes, S., Smith-Merry, J. and O'Donovan, M.A., 2024. Ethical Inclusion and Participation of People with Disability in Research: Problematising Vulnerability. In *Advances in Disability Research Ethics* (pp. 71–90). Emerald Publishing Limited.

Smith-Merry, J. (2017). Inclusive disability research. In *Handbook of research methods in health social sciences* (pp. 1–19). Springer, Singapore.

Smith-Merry, J., 2020. Evidence-based policy, knowledge from experience and validity. *Evidence & Policy*, *16*(2), pp.305–316.

Szucs, B. and Harpur, P., 2023. Students with Disabilities as Ideal Graduates: Universities' Obligations to Support Extracurricular Involvement. *Journal of Teaching and Learning for Graduate Employability*, *14*(2), pp.33–53.

Watharow, A., 2021. *'Not knowing what is going on': The experiences of people with deafblindness–dual sensory impairment in Australian hospitals—a mixed methods study* (Doctoral dissertation, University of Technology Sydney (Australia)).

Index

ableism. 8, 12, 14, 18, 33, 122, 147, 249

academic outcomes. 240

accessibility. 94, 107, 109, 111, 112, 113, 114, 115, 130, 135, 139, 140, 141, 243, 253, 257

accessible information. 93, 94, 95, 96, 106, 108, 109, 110, 111, 112, 114, 115, 118

accommodation. 19, 20, 55, 56, 67, 71, 78, 83, 94, 215

advocacy. 12, 23, 65, 72, 133, 134, 203, 209, 240, 253

Article 21. 109

Article 9. 109

atypical linguicism. 95, 103, 105, 106, 108

autism. 36, 62, 64, 75, 86, 88, 89, 90, 203, 205, 206, 207, 209, 212, 213, 214, 215, 217, 219, 220, 223, 224, 228, 229, 230, 231, 232

Autistic community. 209

codesigned. v, x, 4, 5, 13, 19, 20, 23, 26, 27, 31, 59, 62, 74, 80, 81, 82, 227, 265

communication style. 75, 226

consultation. 75, 76, 156, 211, 219, 223, 229, 237, 245, 248, 259

Convention on the Rights of Persons with Disabilities (CRPD). 109, 157, 236

co-occurring conditions. 75, 130

co-produced. 12, 13, 19, 20, 26, 147, 148, 223, 227, 265

Co-produced policy. 25, 26

data collection. 127, 136, 222, 261

deafblindness. 121, 123, 124, 125, 132, 133, 145, 152, 154, 156, 157, 158, 267

Department of Social Services. 89, 134, 150

depression. 131, 212, 216

descriptive statistics. 78

Diagnostic and Statistical Manual of Mental Disorders fifth edition. 213

disability hiring. 259

disability policymaking. 2, 23, 26

disability services. 3, 30, 33, 57, 61, 111

disability studies. 4, 9, 21, 22, 27, 32, 35, 74, 228, 252

disclosing. 239

double empathy problem. 215, 231

dual sensory impairment. 5, 121, 132, 133, 134, 143, 145, 151, 152, 154, 157, 159, 265, 267

Easy English. 95, 109, 111, 115, 116, 119

Easy Read. 109, 110, 111, 112, 115, 117

epistemic injustices. 122, 123, 136, 137, 142, 149

epistemology. 136, 149

funding streams. 252

generalised anxiety disorder. 212

global disability. 127

hearing loss. 98, 99, 124, 127, 128, 129, 133, 145, 158

human rights. 1, 9, 23, 32, 69, 82, 94, 108, 124, 145, 202, 209, 238, 262, 266

Indigenous population. 128

information deprivation. v, 5, 93, 94, 95, 98, 100, 103, 113, 114, 265

inherent knowledge. 220

insider research. 207, 219, 222, 225

intellectual disability. 15, 34, 55, 64, 65, 66, 67, 68, 75, 89, 91

International policies. 132

language discrimination. 97, 103

leadership. 11, 19, 32, 236, 239, 243, 244, 250, 252, 259, 262, 266

linguistic assimilation. 104

literacy. 94, 95, 96, 98, 103, 104, 106, 107, 112, 113, 114, 115, 137

low literacy. 94, 95, 96, 97, 104, 107

medical model of disability. 99, 204, 240

mental health. 8, 9, 29, 32, 35, 58, 59, 60, 62, 70, 79, 81, 85, 87, 88, 90, 91, 92, 151, 153, 212, 231

National Disability Insurance Scheme. 8, 134, 150

neurodivergence. 12, 18, 22, 201, 202, 203, 205, 207, 208, 210, 216, 217, 227

neurodivergent. 5, 12, 13, 18, 19, 25, 33, 36, 202, 203, 204, 205, 207, 208, 211, 212, 215, 227

non-disabled researchers. 240, 256

operant conditioning. 206

oppression. 106, 145, 205

participatory research. 58, 79, 203, 208, 223, 224, 225, 226, 227, 229, 232, 233

Participatory research. 72, 222, 225

partnerships. 20, 222, 247, 251, 255, 257

Plain Language. 109, 111, 120

policy frameworks. 74, 132

policymaking. 60, 71, 73, 82, 83, 147, 203, 209

policy objectives. 208

qualitative research. 9, 31, 36, 79, 208, 225

queer theory. 98

reflexivity. 208, 225

research participation. 75, 242, 260

research process. 4, 22, 75, 208, 220, 236, 243

research systems. 252

research topics. v, 5, 26

Restrictive practices. 56, 67, 82, 87, 89, 91

seclusion. 58, 59, 62, 76, 82, 84, 85, 86, 87, 88, 89

sensory impairment. v, 123, 129, 132, 146, 153, 155, 158

Signing. 102

social participation. 95, 96, 99, 102, 104, 113, 114, 115, 154, 157

stigma. 2, 7, 72, 89, 107, 122, 143, 210, 214, 216

system deficits. 257

tokenism. 223, 252

underdiagnosis. 127

university policies. 238

university strategy. 241

visual impairment. 128

women with disabilities. 201

www.ingramcontent.com/pod-product-compliance
Lightning Source LLC
Chambersburg PA
CBHW072127190326
41534CB00029B/759
* 9 7 8 1 9 1 8 0 2 6 0 3 0 *